PROFESSIONAL ISSUES IN PRACTICAL/VOCATIONAL NURSING

Delmar Publishers' Online Services

To access Delmar on the World Wide Web, point your browser to:

http://www.delmar.com/delmar.html

To access through Gopher: gopher://gopher.delmar.com

(Delmar Online is part of "thomson.com", an Internet site with information on
more than 30 publishers of the International Thomson Publishing organization.)

For information on our products and services:

email: info@delmar.com

or call 800-347-7707

PROFESSIONAL ISSUES IN PRACTICAL/VOCATIONAL NURSING

Lois Harrion, MS, RN
Independent Trainer in Human
    Resource Management

Director of Vocational Nursing
Simi Valley Adult School
Simi Valley, California

Provider of Continuing Education
    for Nurses
L'MARCA Consulting & Associates
Camarillo, California

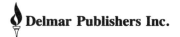 Delmar Publishers Inc.

NOTICE TO THE READER

Delmar Staff

Associate Editor: Marion Waldman
Editing Supervisor: Marlene McHugh Pratt
Production Coordinator: Helen Yackel
Design Supervisor: Susan C. Mathews

For more information address
Delmar Publishers Inc.
3 Columbia Circle Box 15-015
Albany, New York 12212-5015

Printed in the United States of America
Published simultaneously in Canada
by Nelson Canada,
a division of The Thomson Corporation

10 9 8 7 6

Library of Congress Cataloging-in-Publication Data
Harrion, Lois.
    Professional issues in practical/vocational nursing/Lois Harrion.
        p. cm.
    Includes index.
    ISBN 0-8273-3680-2
    1. Practical nursing.   I. Title.
    [DNLM: 1. Nursing, Practical.   WY 195 H312p]
    RT62.H33   1992
    610.73′06′93—dc20
    DNLM/DLC
    for Library of Congress   91-28187
                                                            CIP

Dedication

This work is dedicated to ... my husband Milton, for his technical assistance
my daughter, Karma, for her belief in me
my friend Betty, who teaches me courage

Contents

Preface

This book was prepared for students in education programs for practical/vocational nursing. The ten chapters will include a variety of subject matter and information to provide a foundation for the student entering contemporary practical/vocational nursing.

Discussions on student life will help the student adjust to new roles and responsibilities. A study of the historical perspectives of nursing provides an awareness of the foundation of nursing. Nurturing strategies and self-care for the care-giver remind us of the importance of maintaining a healthy balance between our professional and personal lives. Technological advancement and the changing and expanding role of the practical/vocational nurse require a study of ethical and legal issues. For some issues, there are no clear-cut answers and solutions, and many questions are likely to remain unanswered. Continuing education, maintaining currency of practice, goal setting, and networking are discussed. The chapter on career awareness includes important steps and procedures involved in securing the right job. Suggestions on preparing for the NCLEX-PN licensure examination are included. Leadership, role responsibilities, and organizations are presented. A review of the various kinds of healthcare settings, levels of care, and nursing care delivery methods will help the student better understand how health care is delivered.

CHAPTER
1

Student Life

The student successfully attaining the goals of this chapter will be able to:

- List course subjects that are included in practical/vocational nurse training programs.
- Identify the skills necessary to time-manage activities.
- Describe specific time wasters with possible solutions.
- Use a note-taking system.
- Organize notes for easy reference and study.
- Describe the process of textbook annotation.
- Identify test-taking guidelines.

Congratulations on your decision to become a licensed practical/vocational nurse. You are entering a program of study that will require your full attention, hard work and dedication.

Some of you may have recently graduated from high school, while others may not have been in a formal educational setting for many years. Being away from the classroom for long periods of time does not mean that learning has not taken place. Informal educational experiences occur in everyday life. Life experiences and responsibilities help create an openness to learning.

Some adult learners may not have developed a personal sense of direction, and their personal and professional goals may not be set. Adult learners returning to school after several years of absence may find it difficult to balance the demands of being a student with personal and family responsibilities. Setting realistic goals for yourself, and a positive attitude will assist in your success!

PROGRAM STRUCTURE

Nursing program orientations are usually held several months before the actual course of study begins. Faculty and administrators are present to welcome you and to provide information about the program and the services offered. Topics may include program regulations, classroom rules, uniform requirements, dress codes, hospital and clinical affiliation rules, and student conduct. Frequently, representatives from various student services will also attend the orientation program. The student services may include the resource center, library, counseling office, job placement center, student loan department, and the health center. A more detailed orientation on the academic requirements, grading, and student performance appraisal system is held during the first few days of the program.

Some programs are twelve months long, others eighteen months. The twelve-month programs require students to attend school full time five days per week. The eighteen month programs are part time programs in which students attend class and/or clinical three to four days per week. These programs are designed so that those students who need to maintain employment during their course of study will have the time to work without interfering with their school schedule. Course subjects include anatomy and physiology, nursing fundamentals, pharmacology, medical-surgical nursing, obstetrics, pediatrics, growth and development, nursing history and trends, professional skills and communication, and nutrition.

It is important to know as much about your program and school as possible. Talk with instructors and learn what they expect from students.

Get their requirements about assignments, written work, verbal presentations, student–teacher relationships, tests, grades, course materials, notebooks, and class participation. Ask your instructors how they feel about the use of tape recorders during class. Some may prefer not to be taped, while others' decision may depend on the course material being presented. Your instructors are there to teach the course subject matter, and the more you know about their preferences, the more easily you can meet the requirements for successful completion of your nursing program.

Some programs provide clinical instruction after the theory portion is completed, while others provide the clinical experience concurrently with the theory. Whatever the arrangement, the purpose of the clinical instruction is to provide an opportunity for practical experience. This is the time to apply what you have learned in the classroom. In many nursing programs, students are assigned to a skilled nursing facility or an intermediate care facility during their first clinical rotation. This assignment may last four to six weeks. These settings allow students to experience the first clinical assignments at a slower pace.

During nursing fundamentals, you learn how to plan your clinical day. This plan is in writing and is based upon your patient's diagnosis and condition, physician and nursing orders, and hospital requirements. Your instructor is there to help you in this process. Some skills require instructor observation, while others may be assigned independently without observation. The clinical instructor will determine these requirements.

At the start of the clinical day, you may be expected to go directly to the assigned unit, get a report, and start your patient care. Some instructors prefer to have the students meet for a few minutes before going to the assigned units. Always be prepared to write down pertinent information about your patients. You should be able to answer questions regarding patient care and activity requirements. Your patient assignments are prepared by your instructor in collaboration with hospital personnel. Breaks can be scheduled or you may be expected to schedule with other students. This allows students to monitor each other's patients during the absences. During the day, be sure to seek assistance when needed. You are not expected to step outside your student role in making decisions, and you are expected to seek assistance when physical demands are beyond your abilities.

Postconferences are held at the end of the clinical day. Topics may be assigned to students for presentation, or the instructor may provide speakers, video programs, or practice sessions on various topics. Sometimes students are asked to present an interesting or challenging patient case. When this is done, all patient identification is withheld to protect patient confidentiality. You are expected to participate in postconferences and to take notes as appropriate. This is a part of the clinical learning experience.

Knowing the student's role and responsibilities can be an asset to you. You have the responsibility for your learning, and learning is an active process. Instructors and others are guides or facilitators of learning, but the student must be open and receptive. Students are expected to be self-motivated and focused. As a student nurse, you will be constantly evaluated by your instructors and perhaps by some of the hospital nursing staff. Welcome the evaluation process. This is how you discover in which areas you need to focus more time and attention. Grades are important because there is a minimum requirement for successful completion of your nursing program and the state board examinations. However, it is equally important to focus on the questions answered incorrectly, so that you can correct your mistakes and increase your understanding.

Participation in self-evaluation is a learning experience. As a student you must learn to view yourself objectively. This will assist you in learning to be open to constructive evaluation of your clinical performance. It is important to remember that your performance, and not you as a person, is being evaluated. This will help to prevent negative feelings. As you participate in self-evaluation, you will become aware of your strong areas and of those areas needing more work. Choose one weak area, determine what should be done to improve it, and then start to work. An effective way to start self-evaluation is to compare your actions with the expected results. Using expected results as a guide promotes consistency in the evaluation process.

MANAGING YOUR TIME

When you have many important things to do and too little time to do them, you have to decide how to concentrate your energies. Most of us think that time problems are all caused by external things such as the telephone, visitors, and interruptions. In almost all cases, it is possible to influence, if not control, externally caused time management issues. More difficult to identify, as well as to manage, are internally caused time management issues, such as procrastination, indecision, a lack of self-discipline, the inability to say no, the inability to delegate or ask for help, and acting without thinking.

Time is a constant that cannot be changed. So we cannot manage time itself; we can, however, manage our activities relative to time. The skills needed are the ability to plan, organize, ask for help or delegate, and direct. Time management is self-management. Managing our activities relative to time does not mean working harder, just smarter. You must think ahead about what you want to do, and how and when to do it.

Everyone has the same amount of time; some just use it more effectively than others, gaining the greatest results in the shortest period of time.

There are many elements involved in successful management of activities relative to time. All of them cannot be dealt with in this text, but studies have shown that the most important elements are planning, asking for help or delegating, and controlling the lack of self-discipline. Planning will be explored here along with some time management "to do's."

Some time wasters along with possible causes and solutions are also listed in the section on planning.

Planning

Planning answers the basic questions: Where am I now? Where do I want to be? And how do I get where I want to be? You must first evaluate your current situation, then set realistic goals, and finally develop an outline or plan for action. Suggestions may include:

- Determine what it is you want or need to accomplish; think in terms of results, not just activities.
- Make a list of everything involved. At this point you may want to consider asking for some help with various tasks. If so, include who is responsible.
- Assign an expected date of completion for each item, and move it up by several days. For example, you want something completed by September 1; move the date up to August 24th or 25th. This provides for any unexpected issues that might cause an unforeseen delay.
- Next, try to determine the approximate amount of time each item will require for completion. This permits easier handling when you are trying to schedule various activities.
- Based on the expected date of completion, each item can now be placed on the calendar. This is the beginning of a daily "to do" list. As you are placing these items on the calendar, remember not to overload yourself; one to two items per day is sufficient. The activities of day-to-day living will continue and must be considered when scheduling your time for goal-oriented activities.

There are some attractive features outlined here. First, goals are written down, which for some of us provide the basis for a commitment. Second, time lines are established with a built-in solution for possible delays, and the amount of time involved for each step of the process is approximated. As you go about your daily routine, completing the items on your "to do" list, at least one, maybe more depending on the amount of time involved for each item, will be an item needed to complete a goal. Thus reaching goals becomes a reality.

Time Wasters and Solutions

TIME WASTER	POSSIBLE CAUSES	SOLUTIONS
Lack of planning	Inability to see the benefit	Recognize that planning takes time.
Lack of priorities	Lack of goals	Write down goals and the steps involved.
Haste	Lack of planning ahead	Take time to plan.
	Attempting too much in too little time	Attempt less and ask for help.
	Responding to the urgent	Distinguish between the urgent and the important.
Overcommitment	Confusion in priorities; refusal to set priorities	Say no. Put first things first.
Lack of asking for help	Fear that others will not do it your way	Allow for mistakes and do not expect or require perfection.
Indecision	Fear of mistakes; lack of a decision-making process	Use mistakes as a learning tool. Get information and set goals. Check all options and the consequences; make the best decision and go with it.
Visitors	Enjoyment of socializing	Learn to say no. Set time limits for visits.
Telephone	Enjoyment of socializing; inability to say no	Set time limits for calls. Learn to say no.

LEARNING RESPONSIBILITIES

Listening

Listening is an important skill that you will need throughout your career. You will need to learn effective listening skills early in your student life. Listening is an active, conscious process, and it is important to focus on the speaker so that you can hear what is being said.

Taking Notes During a Lecture

Studies and surveys have shown that most students forget at least fifty percent of what they heard just one hour before. It is impossible to remember everything, but it is important to be able to recall significant information. Note taking should capture key information and provide a good basis for studying for tests and various assignments. A significant benefit, of course, is better grades. Additionally, notes should help you determine what your instructor emphasized and focused on during the lecture. Note-taking will also help you remain focused during the lecture and prevent "mind wandering."

There are varying opinions about how to take notes and about the kind of paper to use. If you have a system that works well for you, do not change it. Choose a system that fits your individual style and comfort. Many educational experts suggest using plain, white, lineless paper so you do not have to worry about staying within the lines. Write only on one side of the paper. Later when you are studying, you will not have to

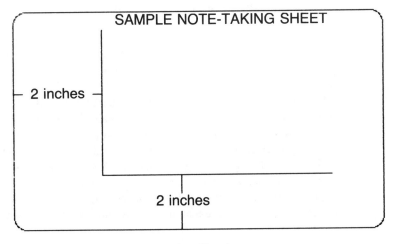

SAMPLE NOTE-TAKING SHEET

2 inches

2 inches

Figure 1-1   Sample Note-taking Sheet

flip pages. The other side of the paper can be used for definitions or additional important notes if necessary. At the top of the page, write the date, subject, and the page number. About two inches from the left edge of the paper, draw a vertical line down the page. Draw another line across the page about two inches from the bottom. These will provide margins for note-taking later. Use two inexpensive folders for each subject, one for class and one for storage of your notes at home. These folders should be labeled with the subject and your name.

When taking notes, just write down everything that is said, do not try to evaluate for importance. You lose time trying to determine what is most important to write down. What you want to do is just process, or write the information. Do not try to outline your notes at this time unless the instructor provides an outline sheet for you. Outlining can be done later.

During study time, or as soon as possible, put in the the's, and's, if's, and other words that will help make sense of the sentences and phrases written. It is important to do this on the same day so that your memory is as fresh as possible. If necessary, see the instructor or a classmate for clarification. Next, try to determine what the important subjects or topics are in your notes, and put Roman numerals beside them in the left margin. You may need to write a two- to three-word title in the left margin. This will help later when you are studying for essay quizzes and tests.

It is estimated that seventy percent of test questions deal with definitions or vocabulary, twenty percent deal with proper nouns and capitalized words, and ten percent deal with numbers—dates, steps, phases, parts, etc. In the bottom margin, list dates, proper names, numbers, capitalized words, definitions and vocabulary words. Now this sheet of paper can be used for studying, because it highlights all the important information on that page. Titles have been noted in the lefthand margin and key words have been written in the bottom margin. The lefthand margin notes can be used when studying for essay tests, and the bottom margin notes can be used when studying for multiple choice, fill-in-the-blanks, or listing test questions.

During the lecture, be sure to take note of anything the instructor writes on the chalkboard. This information is usually important. Sometimes instructors will use key phrases such as, ''now this is important,'' or ''let me give you an example of what I mean,'' ''this will be on the test,'' or ''you will see this again.'' These phrases are good indications of what the instructor considers important. You can also check the amount of notes taken on a particular subject. If you have a large amount of notes on a subject, this may indicate that the topic is important and could generate several test questions.

Textbook Annotation

Textbook annotation is the process of emphasizing key elements of information in the book. It will assist you in studying and preparing for quizzes and tests. Reading is a process that requires active participation. When we read, we need to remain focused on what we are doing to obtain meaning from the words.

First, get an overview of the chapter you are reading. Read the introduction to determine what the author hopes to accomplish, the goals, and the varied items to be discussed. Next, check the summary, if one is included. This usually tells what goals were accomplished. Textbooks are usually written from an outline with the major divisions of the chapter in bold type. Assign Roman numerals to the major subject divisions and capital letters to the subdivisions. When reading, set a goal for yourself before taking a break. Concentrate on that particular section and avoid all interruptions. The margins will provide space for annotations. Underline or highlight the topic sentence of each paragraph. This sentence may or may not be the first sentence. If the paragraph contains only one sentence, then highlight only the key words. When you come across definitions, write the word defined in the left margin, bracket the definition in the paragraph, and draw an arrow to connect the two. When you bracket the definition, do not include the word defined. Write dates in the left margin, using the brackets to show the purpose and the arrow to connect.

When studying for tests using the textbook annotations, the following suggestions may help:

1. Read the topic sentence.
2. Look at the words in the left margin, test yourself on the bracketed information. If you do not get the answers correct, mark an X beside the word. When you review again, you will know where to focus your time and energies.

Studying and Test Taking

Whether you study alone, with a "study buddy," or with a group, choose the situation that best suits your style and meets your needs. Good study habits are essential if you are to complete your academic goals. The amount of time devoted to studying will be determined by the number of subjects in your schedule. It is important to schedule your time for study on a regular basis. Many students determine the amount of time for each subject based on the difficulty of the material. Others suggest studying the more difficult material and the most important subjects first. Many students find it necessary to study every day for a set period, while others study four to five days per week three to four hours per day. Find a schedule that best suits your lifestyle and needs. You may choose to study at home or at the library, but find a place with a minimum of distractions and good lighting. Be sure to have all materials, notes, and books with you to utilize your time efficiently. To maintain concentration and prevent tiredness, take rest periods at least every hour, and try not to study when you are tired or not feeling well. When possible, you can review notes before and immediately after class.

Once you have a regularly scheduled study time, be committed to it. When necessary, manage interruptions and unscheduled events quickly and efficiently.

Taking Tests

Most students do not enjoy taking tests and quizzes, but they are a part of a student's life. The key to success is to be prepared. Study and note review are essential. "Cramming" the night before or the morning of a test is of little benefit.

Suggested guidelines for test taking include:

1. Know the subject(s) included on the test.
2. Make sure you understand the directions before the test begins.
3. Find out if you will lose points for guessing answers.
4. Be sure to be on time, in your chair, with all necessary materials.
5. When answering multiple choice questions, answers with absolute and qualifying words such as always, forever, only, more, most, least, first, and probably are generally incorrect.
6. Eliminate incorrect options.
7. Look for priority word clues, such as first or second.
8. Select the best answer that you understand.
9. Take the question at face value, do not read into the question.
10. Spend approximately a minute on each question. This does not apply to essay questions.
11. Pace yourself so that you can complete the test.
12. For lengthy passages, read the stem of the questions to determine what information you are looking for.
13. Try to answer every question.
14. Do not challenge questions. This only raises your emotional level and distracts your energy and focus.
15. When you finish, close the test booklet, turn the paper over, or hand it in to the instructor.
16. Most importantly, if you studied, trust yourself. Do not change answers back and forth. Most often, the first answer chosen is the correct one.

Using the Library

Many students returning to school may be out of touch with their library. The library is an excellent resource for study, research materials, current magazines, medical reference books, and (with some larger libraries) research services. The librarian is willing to order materials from other libraries when needed.

The card catalogue is the heart of the library. All materials are listed here by subject matter and by author. Most libraries have their card catalogues on a computerized system that is easy to use. The directions for use are simple and are printed in easy steps on the front of the machine. Materials are coded and numbered. The catalogue number is used to locate the book on the shelves. Some libraries' card catalogues consist of index cards. Two files are maintained; one file lists the books by the subject or title, and the other one lists books by authors' names. The cards include the catalogue number of the books. The books also have the catalogue number and are grouped on the shelves accordingly. The librarian and the librarian assistant will assist you if needed.

All libraries have reference materials that cannot be removed from the library, but, you can copy the information if necessary. Usually coin-operated copying machines are available for your use. Your instructors will expect you to access current information for your various nursing assignments. The library offers a wide variety of materials including magazines and journals from professional and student nursing organizations. These references will prove invaluable to you in your studies and in your professional nursing career.

REVIEW/DISCUSSION/ACTIVITIES

1. List the skills required to manage activities relative to time.
2. Identify a time waster in your life. Develop a plan toward a solution and discuss in a class discussion group.
3. Review the section on taking notes during a lecture and discuss those techniques you find helpful.
4. Develop a study schedule. What personal adjustments were necessary in developing this study schedule?

BIBLIOGRAPHY

Macdonald-Clark, N. "Time Management for Nurses Returning to School." *Home Healthcare Nurse* (1983).

Morgan, C. T. *How to Study*. New York: McGraw-Hill, 1989.

Pauk, W. *How to Study in College*. Boston: Houghton Mifflin, 1984.

Lenier, W., and Maker, J. *Keys to College Success*. Englewood Cliffs, N.J.: Prentice-Hall, 1980.

CHAPTER

2

Taking Care of Yourself

The student successfully attaining the goals of this chapter will be able to:

- List three factors that influence personal health.
- Describe several personal actions that contribute to emotional well-being.
- Identify eight factors that help to improve verbal communication.
- Describe the steps in problem-solving.

As health care practitioners, nurses must accept responsibility for personal appearance. They are responsible for the maintenance and preservation of health and the well-being of others. This is a full-time job, and nurses frequently leave themselves to the very last and all too often pay no attention to their own personal and emotional needs. This section will provide some strategies to assist you in taking care of yourself.

PRESENTING A POSITIVE IMAGE

Schools of nursing have dress codes and rules about personal appearance. You may feel that it is unnecessary to discuss such personal issues as bathing, using deodorant, wearing clean clothes and hose, and polishing shoes. There are very specific reasons that these issues are discussed. The image you project leaves a lasting impression on your patients. They take that image with them when they leave the hospital, and they may even discuss it with people in the community. If the image projected is not a positive one, it could be damaging for you and for the hospital. Besides, it will damage the confidence the patient has in you as a professional.

Daily bathing is essential, to prevent odor and the buildup of bacteria on the skin. Some people who bathe daily and use deodorant and antiperspirant still experience an unpleasant odor. See your doctor if this is a problem; there are tablets containing chlorophyll that are helpful in treating this. Sometimes there are other reasons for the body odor— washing compounds, bleaches, and various synthetic fabrics. If the clothing fabric is the problem, you may have to discard it. Some synthetic fabrics are not soil-release-treated, and this may be the cause of the odor. The uniform shop may be able to suggest some special type of cleaner or odor remover, or your local dry cleaning store may know of an appropriate product.

Using underarm deodorant and antiperspirant will help keep personal body odor in check. The deodorant helps control odor, and the antiperspirant helps prevent perspiration. Some products are designed to control odor and perspiration. Your choice is based on your personal need. If you have sensitive skin or cannot find a product to meet your needs, your pharmacist or your physician may be able to help you.

Frequent dental hygiene is a part of personal care that should not be neglected. Halitosis (bad breath) can result from inappropriate dental and oral care. Brushing and flossing after each meal is recommended. When this is not practical, at least twice daily is suggested. Many dentists recommend the use of an antiplaque toothpaste and oral rinse. Some dental hygienists will recommend chewing gums that are antiplaque and breath-freshening and do not promote tooth decay. When brushing the teeth, partial or dentures, the tongue and the inside of the cheeks should be cleaned very gently with a toothbrush and water. Germs that cause bad breath can be found in the coating on the tongue.

The hair should be clean and well managed. Many nursing schools and hospitals require that hair be worn up off the collar and pulled away from the face. The neatness of your appearance is enhanced, of course, and it is much more sanitary when working with patients. When performing procedures and administering treatments, the hair should not be falling down around the shoulders and perhaps obstructing your vision. Hairs may fall into the sterile dressing field or the patient's wound and thus become a source of infection and contamination.

Long fingernails can be a source of germs, so as a student nurse you are encouraged to wear your nails short with a clear polish. The short length makes it easier to clean under the nails with each handwashing. Nail polish is discouraged, because if the manicure is not well kept, the scratches in the polish are unsightly and can be a good resting place for various germs. Proper handwashing is required. You are taught the correct handwashing procedures in your nursing program and are expected to continue the practice. In fact, many programs will evaluate you on the frequency and the correctness of the procedure.

While you are a student, the school will expect you to wear the school uniform and follow the dress code. As a graduate seeking a job, you may expect healthcare agencies to have a dress code. Many do not require their nurses to wear caps, but some nurses still prefer to wear their nurse's cap. These nurses say that they worked very hard to earn the cap and consider it to be a part of their uniform. Others say that patients have commented that the cap adds a look of professionalism and helps make no mistake about who the nurse is.

Your appearance says a lot about how you feel about yourself. It can be interpreted that if you feel good about yourself, then you will feel good about others. The uniform dress and pants should be an appropriate length. The styles of uniforms available are numerous, but there are some things to consider when making your choices: appropriate length, fit, professional look, convenience, and ease of care. Uniforms that fit snugly and are revealing may promote inappropriate patient behavior. Undergarments should be free of designs; beige is the color choice since it has proven to be less revealing, and undergarment lines will not readily be seen.

The feet are very often neglected. Good foot care includes properly fitting shoes, daily cleansing, lubrication and moisturizing, trimmed toenails, and foot powders or deodorant shoe powders. Properly fitting shoes will probably be an expensive investment, but a necessary one. Your shoes should preferably be made of leather and designed for walking. Because you spend a significant amount of time on your feet, the type of shoes you wear will affect your legs, ankles, and back. Shoes should be polished every other day and cleaned once weekly or as often as needed. A soft, dry, clean cloth can be used for buffing after the shoe polish is dry. Foot hose is necessary. If you cannot wear nylon hosiery, then white socks are appropriate. Check with your instructor regarding dress code. If your shoes require shoelaces, be sure to purchase an extra pair so you will always have clean ones to use while laundering the other pair.

When choosing fragrances, makeup, and jewelry, remember: "light" is the word. Your patients will appreciate it. Makeup should be applied lightly and appropriately. Fragrances should never be heavy, oil-based products. A pleasant, clean, nonlingering scent is appropriate. There are some areas of the hospital in which wearing fragrance is not recommended, such as one-day surgery, diagnostic laboratories, cardiology laboratory, surgery, and recovery room. Your jewelry should be limited to small post earrings, your watch, and a plain band. Rings with stones are to be avoided because the stone settings can harbor bacteria, scratch your patients while you are giving care, get caught on various objects and cause injury, and become lost.

PERSONAL WELLNESS

Paying attention to your physical and emotional health is important. As a nursing student you are facing many new responsibilities and tasks, and the demands can be taxing. When you are healthy, it is easier to take care of your patients and carry out your assignments. Your personal health is your responsibility, it is in your control, and it is your choice. You must pay attention to yourself consistently to maintain optimum personal health.

Taking on these additional activities may tax your energy level and cause you to be more tired than usual. The additional hours of study and school work will deplete your energy even more. Make time in your busy schedule for additional rest as needed. You will know how much sleep you need, and your body will signal if sleep is neglected. You may notice a lack of mental alertness, feeling tired, irritability, an "I don't care attitude," and forgetfulness.

Your instructor will tell you that it is important to take your scheduled rest breaks. They take you away from your busy schedule, give you an opportunity to sit quietly and reduce your mental and physical pace, and help maintain your stamina during the day.

Some nursing programs will have gyms or health rooms available for exercise. Participate in some form of exercise for good health maintenance. There are many choices of exercise: running, aerobics, muscle strengthening, bicycling, floor exercise, walking, weight lifting and swimming. Many people think that because they are on their feet working every day, their bodies are being exercised. The internal parts of the body, however, are being neglected. Before beginning any kind of exercise program, be sure to check with your doctor. There may be a health issue, and a special program can be designed for you. Whatever exercise program you choose, it must be consistent in order to provide good body and muscle tone, maintain high energy levels, and in some cases help control your weight. Maintaining your internal conditioning is an important part of presenting a positive external image.

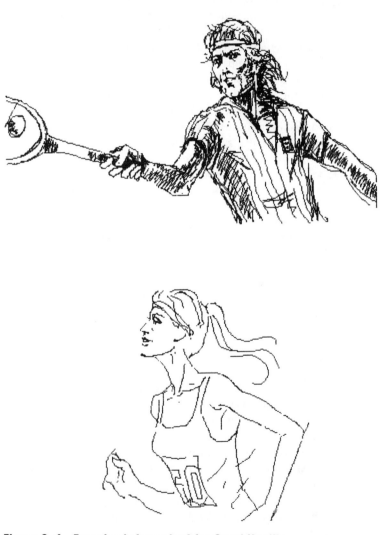

Figure 2–1   Exercise is Important for Good Health

NUTRITION AND DIET

As a nursing student, your schedule will be demanding and fast paced. You may become a prime candidate for "eating on the run" or "I'll just grab something quick." Remember, your performance is affected by what you eat or don't eat. During your course of study, you will learn the importance of good nutrition, the four food groups, and the relationship between good health and good eating habits.

In preparing your eating regime, use the four basic food groups as a guide. In your study of nutrition and diet therapy, you will learn the importance of choosing foods low in saturated fat, salt, sweeteners and cholesterol, and foods high in the complex carbohydrates and fiber.

The most important meal of the day is breakfast. It gets your day off to a good start and helps maintain your energy level through the morning. You will have to plan your meals according to the shift you are working. For example, if you work the night shift, your last meal of the day is breakfast for someone else. Nutritional experts tell us that we need three good, balanced meals. The last meal of the day should be lighter in calories than breakfast and lunch.

Avoid high sugar snacks to provide quick energy. They only provide added calories and do nothing to maintain stamina and alertness. Know what your weight should be for your build, age, and height. Maintain it through exercise and good, balanced nutrition. Maintaining a healthy eating program simply means controlling the amount and types of food you eat. Learn to read the labels on foods to find out about the content.

EMOTIONAL WELL-BEING

Your emotional well-being is directly related to your ability to cope with life issues on a day-to-day basis. The condition of your emotional health is affected by how well you handle the various stressful situations in your life. Maturity is a quality that helps you act responsibly. Nurses must develop relationships with their patients, peers, members of the health-care team, and others. To do so, it is necessary to be receptive to others and to be understanding. Knowing yourself can help you in meeting the emotional demands of nursing.

When you have a reasonable appreciation of your own self-awareness, it is easier to have a healthy respect for others, their opinions, their values, and their beliefs. It is important for nurses to interact well with others. You are expected to create and maintain an atmosphere that promotes positive relationships. That is a part of your responsibility and commitment to nursing.

Self-Care Guidelines

Your emotional health and well-being is just as important as your physical well-being. The demands of your work, the critical decisions you must make, the fast-paced schedules of your personal life, and professional commitments can all take their toll. Nurses are responsible for the maintenance and preservation of health and well-being of others. To do this efficiently, it is important to remember that consistent self-care is necessary. The suggestions listed below are given as basic guidelines to help you learn self-care.

Learn to Say No. Learning to say no can be very difficult. Guilt usually takes over when we say no. But if you don't learn to say no, you will be busy doing things for others and will have no time to do what is important to you. When your help is requested, listen carefully and consider the request. If you can provide the assistance without upsetting your schedule, then say yes. If you can't, then say no. Learning to say no can prevent overburdening yourself with too many tasks, which over a period of time can cause fatigue and illness.

Stop Procrastinating. To help yourself avoid procrastination, make an effort to complete every simple task as soon as it comes your way. When you have a big project, organize it into small, manageable parts. Set aside some time every day or every two or three days to work on a part of the project. Put this time on your calendar and make it a part of your routine schedule. When you complete a small part, reward yourself with a treat. This makes it more appealing to complete the project. The treat can be small and inexpensive, such as a half-hour nap, a coffee or tea break, your favorite television show, or some quiet time to yourself.

Assess Daily Attitudes. Begin to concentrate on those things that matter to you. Arrange your day, week, or month so that you can spend some time doing those things that make you happy. Pay particular attention to the little things that please you, such as browsing through your favorite shop, visiting a flower garden, or eating a meal in the park. Try to start your day with a good thought. Listen to a favorite song or read a meaningful verse or poem. It may take a few extra minutes, but it can be well worth the time.

Provide Adequate Sleep and Nutrition. Frequent abuse of sleep and a lack of a balanced nutritional regime can damage your effectiveness and your health. Listen to the body's signals. Irritability, tiredness, and a lack of mental alertness can mean that your body is saying, "I'm exhausted, take care of me."

Skills for a Healthier Life

There is a difference between "I can't" and "I haven't yet," and you need to learn the skills for acquiring and maintaining a healthier life. Here are some suggestions that might prove helpful.

Stop Putting Yourself Down for Past Poor Habits.   When trying to develop new, healthy habits, make a list of the things you expect to gain from practicing the new habits. Make another list of those things that you must change in order to meet your expected goals. You will quickly see that you can develop a strategy or plan for change when you see what you are up against and what you have to look forward to.

Try Again.   When something doesn't work, learn from your mistakes, and try a different approach. Think of the benefits when the going gets difficult.

Act Like the Person You Want to Be.   Sometimes you may not think about the consequences of growth through the changes you make. The closer your actions come to the perceptions you have of yourself, the more you become what you want to be. For example, you are studying to become a vocational nurse, the more you take on the thinking, the values, knowledge, behaviors, actions, and skills of a vocational nurse, the closer you are to becoming a vocational nurse. Start acting like it has already happened.

Learn to Give Yourself Some Decompression Time.   Take a few minutes or so to step from one role to another. Before beginning your work day, try to forget your personal issues and prepare yourself for the day ahead. At the end of your shift, do the same thing. Don't take your work home, and don't take your home to work.

Do Something Fun Every Day.   If only for a few minutes, make an effort to do something enjoyable. Write it in on your schedule if needed.

Know Your Sore Spots.   Everyone has a weak spot that triggers anger. Once you determine what "pushes your buttons," you can work on decreasing your sensitivity to these sore spots.

Learn to Relax.   When you are involved in a difficult situation, the "fight or flight" syndrome takes over. To counteract this, take slow, deep breaths. Relax your muscles, especially those in the neck, shoulders, and jaw. Keep your voice low, your expression quiet, and your body erect. Not only will you look as if you are in control, you will actually feel calmer. Develop soothing and relaxing habits, such as reading, listening to music, or gardening. Pick an activity that is relaxing for you.

Learn and practice assertiveness.   Assertiveness is the ability to be honest and open when sharing your opinions and ideas. It is a learned behavior and can be expressed through actions and words. Assertiveness shows consistent positiveness through confidence of expression. It does not violate or abuse the rights of others but shows respect for the other person. Assertiveness allows you to remain in control of your emotions and your response to situations. The assertive person:

- will stand up for their own rights without violating the rights of others.
- does not hurt others deliberately.
- listens attentively to the feelings of others.
- reviews personal responsibilities and risks before asserting.
- makes direct statements without excuses.
- uses ''I'' statements in making feelings known.
- remains in control.

KEEPING THE COMMUNICATION CLIMATE HEALTHY _____

Communication is a dynamic, constantly changing process in which there is an exchange of information between a sender or source and a receiver. It is vitally important in nursing. The delivery of patient care is centered on the delivery of information. Communication requires people to interact with one another and, in so doing, respond to messages they receive. It can be accomplished verbally, written or spoken, and nonverbally, through feelings and attitudes.

The components of communication are the sender, the message, and the receiver. One-way communication takes place when the message comes from the sender to the receiver without a response from the receiver. An example of one-way communication is a radio or television broadcast. Two-way communication takes place when the message from the sender prompts a response from the receiver. A conversation between two people is an example of two-way communication.

In the communication process, the sender forms an idea influenced by values, language, knowledge, attitudes, and other factors. The message is sent to the receiver who takes it and transforms it into an idea based on values, language, knowledge, attitudes, and other factors. The effectiveness of communication is dependent upon the mutual understanding of the language and symbols used. Some communication experts say that in order for communication to take place, the sender and the receiver must share a common knowledge and understanding of the language used and the discussion between the sender and the receiver must continue until the message is understood by both, regardless of the words used.

Nonverbal communication is the use of body language for expression. It can be an effective means of communication. Examples include frowning, folded arms, slumped shoulders, silence, facial expressions, posture, gait, and smiling.

In nursing, developing therapeutic nurse–patient relationships is essential. *How* you communicate is as important as *what* you communicate. How you communicate is influenced by your personal style, knowledge, feelings, values, attitudes, opinions, emotions, and age. What you communicate is influenced by your command of the language and symbols being used. Good communication skills include using judgment before you speak, speaking with clarity and confidence, being direct with responses, and being a good listener.

The following suggestions may help to improve verbal communications.

- Think about what you want to say before speaking.
- Face the person you are talking to and use eye contact.
- Use language appropriate to the receiver and the conversation.
- Do not use inappropriate terms such as ''dear,'' ''sweetie,'' etc.
- Use appropriate titles such as Mr., Mrs., Ms.
- Keep your personal opinions and values out of the communication.
- Be a good listener as well as a talker.
- Ask for feedback from the listener to ensure understanding.
- Avoid inferences and sarcasm.
- Seek the listener's level, sit or stand to maintain eye contact.

You must consider factors affecting communication in order to better understand what can help or hinder the communication process. Language barriers are very common when a nurse deals with patients from diverse ethnic and cultural backgrounds. Some healthcare agencies have staff members who may interpret for the patient and the nurse. Other agencies have a list of people who are available to come into the facility and translate on an ''on call'' basis. The inabilty to communicate can be frustrating for the nurse and the patient. It can delay care to the patient or make the patient feel uneasy about care that is given.

The age of the patient will influence the language used and the approach. Children may have a limited vocabulary so the language will have to be at their level of understanding. Pediatric nurses will sometimes draw pictures and use books with stories and pictures to provide assistance in giving information to young children. When working with the elderly patient, a slower pace and less technical language should be used.

Sex can be a factor in the type of information a patient is willing to discuss. For example, the male patient may be more comfortable in discussing intimate issues with a male nurse, and the female patient may prefer to discuss these issues with female nurses.

The educational background of a patient must also be considered. Talking in highly technical and sophisticated terms can leave a disrespectful impression. The message is lost if the patient and family do not understand the language used.

LISTENING

Listening is the interpretive tool used to receive what a person is communicating to you. Good listening skills can be developed, and they affect the communication between you and others. Patients will be more comfortable in talking about their issues with you if they believe you are listening and focused on what they are saying. You can do this by sitting down and maintaining eye contact. This lets the patient know that you can take the time to listen. Sit within an appropriate distance. Provide privacy and a quiet environment by leaving the room door open slightly. Remember, do not impose your ideas, thoughts, attitudes, opinions, and advice. When you are listening to your patients, try not to be judgmental and treat their conversation with confidentiality. To show your interest, you may ask questions relating to the conversation, but don't probe into personal affairs. Your patient may share a story of interest; remain focused and do not try to match their story by telling your own personal story.

When you listen well to the words of others and learn to observe the manners of expression with which the words are conveyed, then you are practicing openness in communication. Finally, respect the right of others to speak, focusing on the message and not on the speaker's style of delivery.

Test on Listening Habits

Do you . . .

1. Act impatient or fidget while others are speaking?
2. Pretend attentiveness, while your mind is elsewhere?
3. Listen selectively, picking out part of the facts and ignoring the whole content?
4. Fail to ask questions when a statement is unclear?
5. Become easily distracted from the conversation?

6. Judge a message unworthy because of the speaker's appearance or delivery?
7. Predict what the speaker will say before it is said?
8. Smother the conversation by making frequent corrections?
9. Spend more time in forming your answer than in concentrating on what is being said?

Some of you will admit to several of these bad habits. Nevertheless, you can become a more effective listener and communicator by becoming attuned to good listening techniques.

PROBLEM SOLVING

Nursing is a rapidly changing profession facing new challenges, trends, and problems every day. Nurses must assume a responsible role in meeting current issues and problems and in anticipating future health needs of our society. An important part of this role is the ability to solve problems and plan effectively.

The most recommended style of problem-solving seeks the best solution and the maximum satisfaction of *all* concerned. Everyone affected must have a vested interest in the outcome and feel that they share the common goal of solving the problem. Effective problem-solving can lead to innovation and energize people to activity.

A Problem-Solving Method

The following is a procedure for planning strategies for problem resolution.

1. Determine what the problem is. Define it in your words.
   Who sees it as a problem?
   Who is affected by it? How are they affected?
2. Get as much information as possible. Make sure that your information is factual and accurate. Use reliable and validated sources of information.
3. Determine the cause of the problem.
4. Decide on the goal or objective. In other words, exactly what it is that you want to do.
5. Examine all the alternatives, including doing nothing. Study each alternative to find out which will have the least negative impact on all concerned. Remember not to include your personal biases and emotions.

6. When you have chosen the best solution to the problem, find out the best way to implement the solution. If this is an issue on the job, there may be rules and policies in effect that may influence the way the solution is carried out. It is important to determine who is most qualified to implement the action.

7. One of the most important steps in problem solving is evaluation. Once you have tried out an alternative, evaluate it to see if this solution is actually the best one chosen. If it isn't, then try another alternative on the list. Remember to write down the evaluation so that if you need to study this problem again, you will know which alternatives did and did not work. It is important to remember that what may work now may not work in the future with the same kind of problem, and what may not work now may work in the future. The problem may be the same, but the issues surrounding it may be very different.

You must remember that every problem is different, even those with some similarities. Each problem must be viewed in light of its own special circumstances, and solutions must be tailored to best meet the needs of everyone involved.

Planning

Planning is an essential part of nursing care delivery and problem-solving. The purpose of planning is to accomplish work in an organized and rational manner. It is the process by which a program is worked out before being put into action. A great amount of detail can be included in the plan, and wide participation can be obtained in its preparation.

Characteristics of Planning

- Planning is thinking of ideas and so is vital as the basis for completing a plan of action.
- Planning is participative. Effective planning involves various individuals and groups who have knowledge and expertise about the issues being presented.
- Planning is anticipatory. Advancements in health care and nursing require the ability to forecast and make judgments. The ability to plan for future needs is essential.
- Planning is continuous. Effective planning is flexible, allowing for changes to meet current and future needs. The act of planning is more important than any one plan. Past and current information is important to nursing planners to facilitate continuous and effective planning.

Planning Phases

The different phases of planning are interrelated and dependent upon each other, but planning does not always take place in sequential and rigid steps. The planning process includes:

1. Defining common purposes and objectives.
2. Identifying issues and concerns.
3. Selecting the people to participate in planning.
4. Collecting and reviewing the information.
5. Evaluating the needs and the available resources.
6. Developing recommendations.
7. Developing a plan of action.
8. Implementing the plan of action.
9. Evaluating and reviewing the progress of actions taken, and implementing continuous planning.

When you are developing a plan of action, several other considerations must be included:

- Selecting leaders and participants for functional tasks.
- Setting a tentative timetable for completion of each step in the plan.
- Estimating the costs involved.

When recommendations have been developed and the priorities have been determined, a definite plan can be developed. Pay strict attention to the following:

- Specifying goals, objectives, and policies for putting recommendations into action.
- The timetable and the phasing of activities.
- Outlining individual responsibility for carrying out the various actions.
- Providing methods for progress evaluation.

Evaluation of the Plan

A plan is acceptable if it accomplishes the following:

1. Reflects the clearly stated objectives.
2. Outlines the procedural steps for putting the plan into action.
3. Can be communicated effectively and allows for appropriate distribution of information about the plan.
4. Is operational, sound and viable, and economically feasible.
5. Represents the group or groups concerned.
6. Allows for alternative courses of action.
7. Appropriately uses human talents, skills, and abilities and material resources.

REVIEW/DISCUSSION/ACTIVITIES _____

1. Discuss two factors influencing your personal health.
2. Identify at least two changes you need to make in support of personal health and well-being.
3. Review the section on emotional well-being. Which suggestions are most valuable to you? How do you plan to include the suggestions?
4. What are some of the factors influencing communication?
5. What can you do to show that you are listening to the person speaking?
6. What are the four characteristics of planning?
7. How do you evaluate a plan for effectiveness?

BIBLIOGRAPHY _____

Gerrard, B.; Boniface, W.; Love, B. *Interpersonal Skills for Health Professionals*. East Norwalk, Ct: Appleton & Lange, 1980.

Hood, G.H., and Dincher, J. R.: *Total Patient Care: Foundations and Practice*. St. Louis: C.V. Mosby, 1988.

Milliken, M. *Understanding Human Behavior*. Albany, N.Y.: Delmar, 1981.

Muldarv, T.W. *Interpersonal Relations for Health Professionals*. New York: Macmillan, 1983.

Sampson, E.E., and Marthas, M. *Group Process for the Health Professions*. New York: Wiley, 1981.

CHAPTER

3

Historical Perspectives

OBJECTIVES

The student successfully attaining the goals of this chapter will be able to:

- Describe the contributions of Florence Nightingale to modern nursing.
- Identify at least five nursing leaders and discuss their contributions to nursing.
- Identify the major historical periods and identify a significant event of that period.
- Name two organizations primarily concerned with practical/vocational nursing.
- Describe the growth of practical nursing from the late 1800s to current times.

Nursing has a very rich history of change and progression, and the growth continues today. Though much of the historical record of nursing is unclear, nursing has been practiced for centuries. Many names have been used to describe someone caring for the sick, including midwife, attendant, and wet nurse. Such people were usually thought to have a special way with the sick, a mothering quality. Much of the care was done in the home, and the practical nurse was the first home health nurse and visiting nurse.

The training of nurses in early times was left to those who were already providing the care. When training programs for practical nurses were established, the academic aspects were limited to homemaking functions. A very positive change for practical nursing has been the establishment of educational requirements. The practical nurse is called the vocational nurse in some states, and the practice of nursing is governed by a practical/vocational nurse board. The L.P.N./L.V.N. administers care under the direct supervision of the registered nurse. The course for the practical/vocational nurse is usually a year. The nursing board requires a certain number of hours, and this requirement is met through the program scheduling at the individual schools.

As you read about nursing history, you can appreciate the importance of being prepared to meet the future challenges of nursing.

NURSING IN PRIMITIVE CIVILIZATIONS

Illness in primitive times was associated with gods, so the medicine man was an important person in the community as the intermediary between the gods and the sick person. Herbs and songs were used for purifying the sick.

Rivers and waterways became the source of life for many of the early civilizations. In Egypt, Apollo was considered the god of medicine, and great temples were built in his honor. These temples were used to house and treat the sick. Egyptian physicians treated fractures and filled teeth. There is little recorded about nursing in these times, though it is known that midwives practiced obstetrics.

The Old Testament of the Bible refers to nursing functions. There was a close relationship between religion and medicine. The priests worked as the health person in charge. The sick houses were places for people with communicable diseases.

Late in the fifth century B.C., Hippocrates (460–370) translated the teachings of the priests into a textbook of medicine. He was called the Father of Medicine and is still referred to by that title today. He is credited with putting the study of medicine on a more academic and scientific level. His textbook removed some of the superstitous beliefs that were practiced. Socrates, Plato, and Aristotle were Greek physicians who believed in the teachings of Hippocrates. They all believed that illness and diseases had definite causes. The Hippocratic oath is still used today as the ethical code of medical practice.

The women in Greece were considered subordinate to men and were not trained in nursing. The men who practiced Hippocratic medicine also performed the nursing functions. The women did the nursing of the children in the household.

NURSING IN THE CHRISTIANITY AGE

The Roman Empire was built on military strength. Military hospitals were built for the wounded soldiers, and the nursing was done by friends or relatives. Roman medicine was not as advanced as Greek medicine. The printed works of Hippocrates could not be read by very many people, so many of his advancements were lost.

With the acceptance and growth of Christianity, nursing was done by women of Christian charity. Later, men and women called deacons and deaconesses practiced charitable nursing. They took care of the needy, the aged, the sick, the homeless, and the poor. The deaconesses were the first to perform as visiting and home health nurses. Phoebe was a deaconess, a practical nurse, and the first visiting nurse. The deacons and deaconesses were ordained by the Church and lived in very simple circumstances. They are frequently referred to as the first public health nurses.

NURSING IN THE DARK AGES AND THE MIDDLE AGES

After years of attacks by the barbarians, Europe split into many kingdoms. The Dark Ages lasted about 500 years, and learning during this time came to a halt. It was a time of war and confusion. Christians lived in the monasteries, and the monks continued to learn and kept a history of the past. The Church directed the care of the sick in the monasteries, and the monks and nuns provided the care. The focus was to provide comfort and personal care. Men and women, the monks and nuns, continued to provide care, and the first nursing orders of nuns were formed.

The Crusades, a series of religious wars, began during the Middle Ages. The Crusaders were military orders of priests, brothers, and knights who were trained to fight as well as take care of the sick. Their purpose was to take back the Holy Land from the Moslems. They built hospitals to care for the sick and injured. One order of monks known as the Knights Hospitalers had as its symbol a red cross, which is now the symbol of the International Red Cross.

Hospices were formed in the monasteries. The popularity of the deaconesses seemed to fade, and the monastery nursing orders replaced them. The hospices were not just for the sick; they also took in travelers and the poor. One of the early monastic orders, The First Order of St. Francis, is still active today. It was founded by St. Francis of Assisi.

The strict nursing orders of the Middle Ages provided some organization to nursing. The members of the orders were expected to be obedient and to live secluded in poverty. They were to provide unselfish service to the needy. Nursing was becoming an acceptable occupation for women. The strength of the nursing orders increased as the Catholic Church grew in popularity and strength. The Church, had direct authority over nursing. The nurse's first order of business was to take care of the patient's spiritual needs. Nursing care during this time was custodial and not medically oriented.

The Crusaders returned to Europe, bringing with them the bubonic plague. The plague was a very contagious disease, and during the 1300s one fourth of the population contracted the disease and died. The economies declined, and at the end of the Middle Ages, religious interest was low. The Church's influence began to decline, and the chaotic times caused a feeling of hopelessness and despair.

NURSING FROM THE RENAISSANCE TO THE NINETEENTH CENTURY

Martin Luther, who opposed the teachings of the Catholic Church during the Reformation founded a new religion, Prostestantism. Many changes took place. Monasteries were closed, religious orders were abolished, and nursing virtually came to a halt. In Prostestantism, women were subordinate to men. The tradition of service to the needy disappeared, and the poor, the homeless, and the sick were neglected.

During the Renaissance, medicine came to the forefront with the study of the sciences. Nursing continued to decline. During this time a French priest, St. Vincent de Paul, founded the Sisters of Charity, a nursing order that took care of the poor and the sick.

Industrialization was strong on the scene in the eighteenth century. There were severe human problems, such as child labor, overcrowding, and poor working conditions. Hospitals could not meet the needs of the people, and at one time the mortality rate for women in labor reached one-hundred percent! Patients who went to the hospital often became more ill than when they were admitted to the hospital.

In 1847, a Hungarian obstetrician, Ignaz Semmelweis, developed and used the first antiseptic methods. He discovered the cause of the fever that was killing the women who had babies in the hospitals. He believed the puerperal fever was given to the mothers by the medical students who came from the autopsy room. At his insistence, physicians washed their hands before caring for the obstetrics patients. Instruments were also washed in a solution of chloride of lime, and the puerperal fever deaths decreased significantly.

In America, the physicians were not trained very well. Nursing was done by a few religious orders and by people who were untrained. The first hospital was built in Philadelphia through the influence of Benjamin Franklin.

The hospitals were inferior. The wards were dirty, and the patients suffered pain, infections, and gangrene. Nursing was not a desirable occupation. People from the criminal segment of society replaced the nurses as careers for the sick. Patients were abused, and drinking on duty was acceptable behavior.

NURSING IN THE NINETEENTH AND EARLY TWENTIETH CENTURIES

Homeless, sick, poor, and insane persons were put in jails, hospitals, and poorhouses. Living conditions were deplorable. The large cities were open doors for poverty and disease. The hospitals did not have sanitary conditions. There was no supervision, and no nursing care was given at night. Perfume was used to cover the odor of the illness and disease.

Theodor Fliedner (1800–1864), a German pastor, opened a school in Germany to train deaconesses. It was called the Kaiserwerth Deaconess Institution. This was considered to be the first nursing school, and the most famous of its graduates, Florence Nightingale, is the founder of modern nursing.

Florence Nightingale was born in Italy of very wealthy parents. She was an attractive, serious young lady with an excellent education in philosophy, languages, mathematics, and history. Florence had a special feeling about nursing and social reform. She objected to the idea that women of culture and prestigious positions should not seek careers. Her family opposed the idea, but she followed her heart. She traveled extensively in England, Egypt, Greece, and France. She wanted to see how nursing was being administered and to learn as much as she could. At the age of 31, she entered the Kaiserwerth Deaconess Institution as a student nurse and spent three months in training.

Florence's first graduate position was in England as the superintendent of the Establishment for Gentlewomen During Illness. In 1853, the Crimean War started, and the British newspapers wrote of the horrible conditions and the poor care being given the British soldiers. Florence was asked by the Secretary of War, Sir Sidney Herbert, to go to the

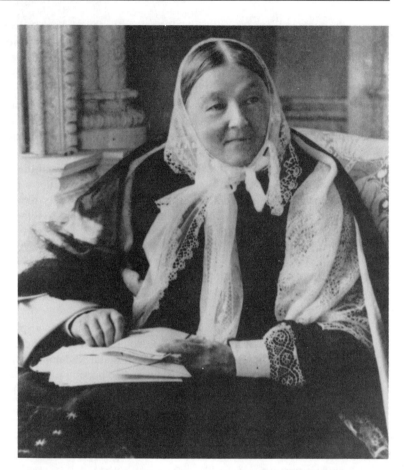

Figure 3–1 Florence Nightingale. *Courtesy The Center for the Study of the History of Nursing.*

Crimea and care for the wounded soldiers. She took with her thirty-eight women, some of whom were trained as nurses, others not. They found the conditions horrible: cholera was epidemic, sanitation was almost nonexistent, the food was bad, and there was no soap or clean linens. The reception by the medical officers was unpleasant. They did not believe that women should be at the front lines.

Florence and the women began to make changes. She organized the nursing care, obtained the needed supplies, set up laundries, and hired people to clean the hospital and provide nourishing meals for the patients. She became known as ''the lady with the lamp,'' as she made her rounds late at night checking on her patients' welfare and comfort.

After her war efforts, she returned to England in 1856. As a semi-invalid, she continued to influence the practice of nursing. She believed that nursing is an art and a science, and she was a strong advocate of nursing education. The Nightingale School opened in 1860 and is considered the first modern school of nursing. Florence was actively involved in research and was a prolific writer. One of the most famous and bestselling textbooks is her *Notes on Nursing: What It is, and What It Is Not*. This book, published in 1859, was written for students and laywomen and has been translated into several languages.

In 1864, the International Red Cross was founded by J. H. Dunant. This organization provided service to nations during wars and after natural disasters. To serve the United States, Clara Barton formed the American Red Cross in 1881.

The United States entered the Civil War in 1861. It lasted for four years with high casualties on both sides. There were no established programs to train nurses. There was opposition, especially in the South, to women working in hospitals. The Civil War showed the need for trained nurses and along with other social conditions was the springboard for developing nurse training schools and programs.

Women's status was improving, and they were taking on new responsibilities in nursing. Bellevue Hospital in New York City opened a training school in 1873, and in 1888 the hospital opened the Mills School of Nursing to train male nurses. Nursing continued to make great strides, and several nursing leaders became prominent.

Dorothea Lynde Dix (1802–1887) was the first U.S. Army Nurse. She worked as an untrained volunteer during the Civil War and eventually was appointed the Superintendent of Women Nurses for all Military Hospitals. She was very concerned about the inhumane treatment of the mentally ill and traveled about the United States to secure the support of legislators for laws to protect the mentally ill.

Clara Barton (1821–1912) took volunteer nursing services to the war area during the Civil War and was known for providing nursing services equally to all soldiers on both sides of the war. For her work during the war, she was given the name "Angel of the Battlefield." In 1881, she founded the American Red Cross and served as its first president.

Linda Richards (1841–1930) graduated from a one year program in Boston as the first trained nurse in the United States. She devoted her professional career to lecturing and organizing nursing services in hospitals throughout the country. As a night superintendent at Bellevue Hospital in New York, she developed a system of making notes on her patients that later became the basis for nursing recordkeeping. Every two years, the National League for Nursing gives the Linda Richards Award to a nurse who has made a significant contribution to nursing.

Isabel Hampton Robb (1860–1910) was one of the first nurses to advocate licensure for nurses as a protection for the patient. She believed in the three-year training program for nurses and devoted efforts to promoting the eight-hour work day for nurses instead of the twelve-hour day. She authored several nursing textbooks and was one of the founders of the *American Journal of Nursing*.

Lavinia L. Dock (1858–1956) was a graduate of the Bellevue Training School and worked as an assistant to Isabel Hampton Robb. She used her knowledge in the establishment of an organization for nursing school superintendents, which is known today as the National League for Nursing. Miss Dock authored the book *History of Nursing*, the classic text on nursing history.

Mary Eliza Mahoney (1845–1926) graduated from the New England Hospital for Women and Children in 1879 as the first African-American Nurse in the United States. She worked as a private-duty nurse, and her work for the acceptance of African Americans in the nursing profession was a lifelong commitment. The National Association of Colored Gradu-

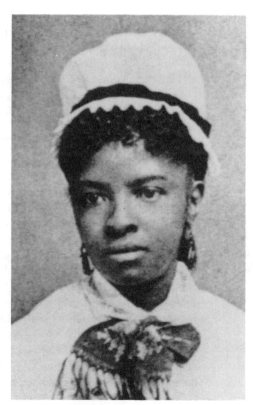

Figure 3–2
Mary Mahoney.
Courtesy Schomberg
Center and The Center
for the Study of the
History of Nursing.

ate Nurses presented the first Mary Mahoney Award in 1936. The American Nurses' Association presents the Mary Mahoney Award biennially to a person who is significantly involved in promoting equal opportunities in nursing for minority persons.

Lillian D. Wald (1867–1940) was concerned about the need for nursing for the poor and opened the Henry Street Settlement in New York City. This was the beginning of public health nursing in the United States. She made contributions to the development of public health nursing and served in 1912 as the first president of the National Organization for Public Health Nursing.

Mary Adelaide Nutting (1858–1947) worked to raise the standards of nursing education and founded the first college-level department of nursing at Columbia University Teachers' College. She coauthored the four-volume *History of Nursing* with Lavinia Dock and was significantly involved in the formation of the International Council of Nurses. The National League for Nursing, during its biennial convention, presents the Mary Adelaide Nutting Award to persons or groups who have made significant contributions to nursing service or nursing education.

Annie W. Goodrich (1876–1955) was an advocate of nursing education and promoted nursing to a professional status. Miss Goodrich

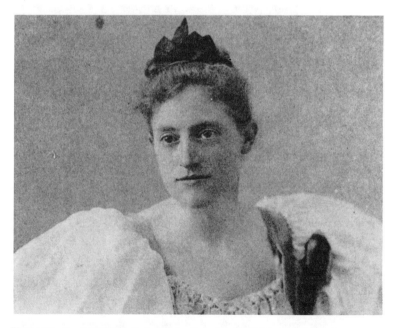

Figure 3–3   Annie W. Goodrich. *Courtesy The Center for the Study of the History of Nursing.*

developed plans for an Army School of Nursing, which earned her the Distinguished Service Medal in 1923. She served as president of the International Council of Nurses, the American Federation of Nurses, the American Collegiate Schools of Nursing, and the American Nurses' Association.

Clara Maass (1876–1901) worked as a contract nurse with the U.S. Army during the Spanish-American War. She volunteered to work in Havana where experiments were being done to discover the cause of yellow fever. She became a test subject and received mosquito bites twice. She recovered from a mild case of yellow fever from the first bite but died ten days after receiving the second mosquito bite. She was the only American and the only woman to die during the experiments. The first stamp issued by the United States to honor an individual nurse was issued in her honor in 1976.

Mary Breckinridge (1881–1965) was a pioneer in nurse midwifery. Miss Breckinridge was from Kentucky and graduated from St. Luke's Hospital in New York. She was instrumental in organizing a Committee for Mothers and Babies in 1925.

Alice Fisher (1939–1988) attended St. Thomas Hospital in London. She was superintendent of several institutions in England, including

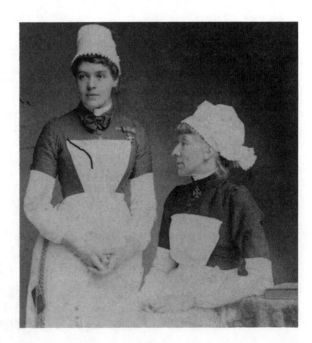

Figure 3–4   Alice Fisher, seated on the right. *Courtesy The Center for the Study of the History of Nursing.*

Fever Hospital in Newcastle, Addenbroke's Hospital in Cambridge, Radcliffe Infirmary in Oxford, and General Hospital in Birmingham. Fisher spent four years in the United States, and during that time, she founded and was superintendent of the Training School for Nurses, as well as chief nurse at Philadelphia General Hospital, Philadelphia. She suffered from a chronic heart problem, but was well known for her hard work, high standards and ideals, and sharp intellect.

Practical/vocational nurses have had various roles in history, depending on the need at the time. They have always been involved in actual nursing tasks. Their beginnings were humble, and many times their efforts went unrecognized. As nursing has increased in status throughout the years, the focus has shifted to nursing education and quality nursing standards. The practical/vocational nurse remains an important member of the healthcare team.

THE GROWTH OF PRACTICAL/VOCATIONAL NURSING ___

In the United States, the Industrial Revolution saw many people leaving the rural areas and moving to the cities. The women who moved to the cities were not educated or trained, and their employment was limited to domestic work.

The first training for practical nurses was offered in 1892 at the YWCA in Brooklyn, New York. The course was three months long, and its primary purpose was to teach practical nurses how to care for the elderly, children, and invalids. Soon after, several schools for training practical nurses were developed. In 1897, the Ballard School, founded by Miss Lucinda Ballard, opened in New York. The Thompson School in Brattleboro, Vermont, was opened in 1907, and in 1918, the Household Nursing Association School of Attendant Nursing was established in Boston. These programs taught home nursing skills, including cooking and nutrition, housekeeping, and simple nursing procedures.

Prior to World War I, the practical nurse was involved in home nursing. By the end of the nineteenth century, practical nursing began to expand from home nursing to public health nursing. Concern for the sick and indigent was regaining public interest.

The early 1900s brought many activities leading to the monitoring of practical nursing. A system for standardization of requirements for practical nursing was developed by the National League of Nursing Education in 1917, but by 1938, New York was the only state with mandatory licensure. Between 1920 and 1940, there were fewer than ten states that had laws to license practical nurses. There were limited controls and very little supervision of practical nursing schools during this period. Much of the work of the practical nurse continued to be in public health nursing and in visiting nurse assignments.

During World War II, preparation began to meet the increased demand for trained nurses. Practical nurses continued to play a vital role, and their employment spread to health departments, industry, and hospitals.

In 1941, the National Association for Practical Nurse Education and Service, Inc. (NAPNES) was formed. It was the first national professional association established specifically for practical nursing. Its membership includes licensed practical nurses, registered nurses, doctors, hospital administrators, students, and public individuals. NAPNES was the first organization to be sanctioned by the Department of Education as an accrediting association for schools of practical nursing. The accrediting service was first offered by NAPNES in 1945; the service was ended in 1984.

During the late 1940s, a committee on practical nurses in nursing service recommended the use of the title "licensed practical nurse." This committee also outlined the differences between the duties of the R.N. and the L.P.N. and specified that the L.P.N. is under direct supervision of the R.N.

In 1949, the National Federation of Licensed Practical Nurses (NFLPN) was founded by Lillian Kuster. This association is the official membership organization for licensed practical and vocational nurses, and membership is limited to L.V.N.s and L.P.N.s.

The National League for Nursing (NLN), set up a separate department for practical nursing programs in 1961. Through this department, schools of practical nursing could be accredited by the NLN. These efforts were supported by the National Federation of Licensed Practical Nurses and by the American Nurses' Association. This elevated practical nursing to a new status because, to be accredited by the NLN, the nursing school had to meet certain standards and criteria, though it is not mandatory for schools to be accredited by the NLN. Approval and monitoring responsibility for practical nursing educational programs is within the authority of the state boards of practical/vocational nursing.

With the nursing shortage, practical/vocational nurses continue to be a vital part of the nursing team. The practical nurse is finding employment in hospitals, clinics, outpatient agencies, visiting nurse agencies, nursing homes, intermediate care facilities, insurance companies, diet and nutritional therapy centers, veterinarians' offices, physician offices, and the military.

REVIEW/DISCUSSION/ACTIVITIES

1. Identify and discuss conditions and events influencing the development of nursing during primitive and early civilizations.
2. Identify some of the personal characteristics of early nursing leaders.
3. Discuss the role of the religious orders in the development of nursing.
4. Discuss the impact of NAPNES, NFLPN, and the NLN on the development of practical/vocational nursing.

BIBLIOGRAPHY

Dolan, J. A. *Nursing in Society: A Historical Perspective.* Philadelphia: W.B. Saunders, 1983.

Donahue, M. P. *Nursing, the Finest Art.* St. Louis: C.V. Mosby, 1985.

Ellis, J. R., and Hartley, C.L. *Nursing in Today's World: Challenges, Issues, and Trends.* Philadelphia: J.B. Lippincott, 1988.

Griffin, Gerald Joseph, and Griffin, Joanne King. *History and Trends of Professional Nursing,* 7th ed. St. Louis: C.V. Mosby, 1973.

Grippando, Gloria M. *Nursing Perspectives and Issues,* 3d ed. Albany, N.Y.: Delmar, 1986.

Saxton D. F.; Nugent, P. M.; and Pelokan P. *Mosby's Comprehensive Review of Nursing,* 12th ed. St. Louis: C.V. Mosby, 1987.

The Nursing Process and The Nursing Team

OBJECTIVES

The student successfully attaining the goals of this chapter will be able to:

- Define the term *patient care team.*
- List the members of the nursing care team and discuss their patient care responsibilities.
- Describe the five steps of the nursing process.
- Identify and discuss four methods of nursing care delivery.

Nursing theories and trends guide the practice of nursing by providing a focus for care of patients. Great emphasis is placed on the whole person and on the participation of the patient in his or her care. Nursing leaders encourage nurses to respect and appreciate all cultures as they practice nursing and administer care to their patients. This respect and appreciation requires adapting nursing care to the needs of patients from various cultures.

THE NURSING PROCESS

The nursing process is a specific way of nursing. It is an organized, systematic method of nursing practice. It requires organization of care delivery so that the patient will receive the optimum benefit. The process includes five steps:

1. *Assessment*—assessing the patient
2. *Diagnosis*—developing the nursing diagnosis
3. *Planning*—planning the nursing care
4. *Implementation*—implementing the nursing care plan
5. *Evaluation*—evaluating the effectiveness of nursing care

The major responsibility for the nursing process belongs to the registered nurse (R.N.). The L.P.N./L.V.N. is not an independent health-care practitioner and always functions under the supervision of the R.N., physician, or dentist. The practical nurse has a vital and active role in all steps of the nursing process except step two, the development of the nursing diagnosis. The judgment and knowledge required to formulate a nursing diagnosis statement are considered to be at the R.N. educational level.

The nursing process can be compared to the problem-solving process described in Chapter Two. In problem-solving, you define the problem, determine what it is you want to do, identify all possible alternatives, choose the most appropriate one, initiate the alternative, and then evaluate the results. The nursing process works in a similar pattern and is the basis of how you administer care to your patients as a student and as a licensed nurse.

Assessment

The assessment phase of the nursing process involves gathering as much information about the patient as possible. This collection of information can be obtained from physical assessment, patient observations, the patient's medical record, and the nursing report. The primary and immediate source of information, when feasible, is your patient. The patient's family can also be of assistance in providing information.

Data gathering and assessment is a continuous process beginning upon admission and continuing throughout the patient's stay. Assessment includes observation, interviewing, and examination. Observation is of the patient's general appearance, personal hygiene, behavior, and physical characteristics. The senses of vision, hearing, touch, and smell can assist in collecting information about the patient's health status. This knowledge base is used to identify the patient's problems. Institutions and agencies have their own forms and formats to be used in the interview process. The L.P.N./L.V.N.'s area of responsibility will be determined by the area of work involved and the institution's policy. During the interview, be sure to let your patient know why you are asking questions and make every attempt to put him at ease. Be a good listener and reassure your patient that he has the right not to answer those questions that make him feel uncomfortable. Listening will require a conscious effort on your part, but it is important to encourage confidence and to put your patient more at ease. Ask for clarification when you don't understand and review statements that concern you: "Excuse me, could you repeat that please?" or "I am not sure that I understand." During the interview process, avoid showing and verbalizing personal disapproval; your responsibility does not include judging the patient's behavior, decisions, or values. If your personal values are involved, it is easy to label the patient. This labeling can prevent the development of an effective therapeutic nurse–patient relationship and so can prevent quality care for the patient.

As you obtain information about your patient you will gather objective and subjective data. Objective information includes the things you can see, such as skin conditions, height, weight, and vital signs. Subjective information is what the patient states or describes, such as a description of symptoms or pain. For example, the patient states he feels warm (subjective); the patient has a temperature of 101°F (objective). It is important to check information for accuracy and to group the information to help identify patterns of illness or wellness. Subjective and objective information are included in the nurses' notes.

The physical assessment is a vital part of the data gathering process. Physical assessment is taught to registered nurses as part of their basic education, but it is a postgraduate course for the L.P.N./L.V.N. The area of employment, agency and institution policy, the level of your additional education, and the acuity of the patient will determine your involvement and responsibility in the patient's physical assessment. You will assist the R.N. with gathering all the data, including laboratory and diagnostic reports and physician information in preparation for formulating the nursing diagnosis. From this information, the R.N. will determine real or potential problems associated with the patient's diagnosis or condition. A differentiation should be made between patient problems and nursing problems. Patient problems are needs of the patient that the nurse may or may not be able to meet. Nursing problems are needs of the patient that can be resolved, changed, or affected by nursing care.

Diagnosis

The second step of the nursing process is formulating a nursing diagnosis. The nursing diagnosis assists in determining the priority of problems for the patient and is the key to individualizing patient care. While this step is the exclusive responsibility of the R.N., you may be asked to provide input in the process, and you will need a basic knowledge and understanding of how it works. Nursing diagnosis is of a real or potential health problem that nurses can provide care for independently by initiating nursing actions (interventions) to reduce, prevent, or resolve the problem. The important question in formulating a nursing diagnosis is, can the nurse independently begin treatment to reduce, resolve, or prevent the problem? When there is a positive answer to this question, then it is correct to formulate a nursing diagnosis.

The North American Nursing Diagnosis Association has developed a list of nursing diagnoses to aid in communication among nurses so that the terminology used is understood by all. The nursing diagnosis statement includes two parts: P for the problem, E for etiology and contributing factors, or cause, identified by using the phrase "related to." Example: "Alteration in Bowel Elimination: Constipation related to imposed bedrest.

The use of nursing diagnosis in the nursing process helps the nurse identify and use information to determine those nursing interventions that will provide maximum benefit to the patient. Figure 4-1 is a care plan using the nursing diagnosis format. The subjective and objective data are included as an illustration of the difference between subjective and objective data. The outcome or goal listed is a long-term goal, and the nursing orders are an example of the nursing interventions that can be applied to this particular nursing diagnosis. These interventions relate very specifically to the nursing diagnosis and provide a possible solution. The possible solutions offered should be moving toward the goal or desired result. Notice that the goal or outcome statement is written positively, as an expectation of what will happen.

Planning

Planning is the third step of thenursing process. It includes determining priorities, developing outcomes or patient-centered goals, determining nursing interventions, and documentation.

Figure 4–1   Nursing Diagnosis/Care Plan (Assessment Phase)

NURSING DIAGNOSIS/CARE PLAN

Nursing Diagnosis	Outcome/Goal	Nursing Orders
Alterations in Bowel Elimination: Constipation Related to Immobility.	The patient will demonstrate improved bowel elimination.	Discuss fluid preferences. Set up a schedule for fluid intake.
Subjective data: Patient reports difficulty; hard dry stools.		Encourage a glass of warm water to be taken ½ hr. ac breakfast.
Objective data: Immobility—traction; forced bedrest.		Assist with bedpan and elevate HOB to high Fowler's if permitted. Provide privacy.

The patient may be admitted with several problems, so it is important to determine which ones are most critical to the patient's welfare. It is possible to work on several problems at the same time, but critical problems should be taken care of first. As the patient's condition changes, the problems may change in severity and priority, so in planning care remember to be flexible.

The patient-centered goals or outcomes indicate problem resolution or desired results. Goals or outcomes must be observable and measurable, and a time frame must be included. When you are writing goals or outcomes, be specific about expectations. The goals/outcomes are for the patient, not the nurse, and they should be attainable. It may be necessary to have a long-term goal and several short-term goals, so the problem can be managed more easily. Short-term goals/objectives are directed toward meeting the long-term goal, but they are smaller and detailed and the time frame is shorter. Short-term goals/objectives can make the problem appear less difficult to resolve because smaller segments of a problem are more easily handled and one can see "a light at the end of the tunnel." Figure 4-2 continues with the care plan used in the previous example. The short-term goals are more manageable parts of the long-term goal. They are stated in smaller, more detailed units to meet the long-term goal. Short-term goals are more detailed and specific, and the nursing orders or actions listed are specific to the short term goals.

When a problem is resolved, it is noted on the care plan. If a problem is not resolved by the date assigned to the problem, then the nursing interventions are discussed and evaluated for appropriateness.

Figure 4–2   Nursing Diagnosis/Care Plan (Planning Phase)

NURSING DIAGNOSIS/CARE PLAN

Nursing Diagnosis	Outcome/Goal	Nursing Orders
Alterations in Bowel Elimination: Constipation Related to Immobility.	Long-Term Goal: The patient will demonstrate improved bowel elimination.	
	Short-Term Goal: Adequate fluid intake of 2 liters per 24 hours. Short-Term Goal: Provide health teaching re: diet	Discuss fluid preferences. Offer fluids every hour and on every visit to patient's room. Keep accurate intake and output record. Discuss dietary preference. Review list of foods high in bulk. Suggest four fruit servings daily. Include moderate use of bran.

The charting system used is determined by each facility. Documentation is necessary, and the written care plan is the guide for documenting the care administered. Charting should reflect that the care plan was carried out and should indicate the patient's responses to the nursing interventions. The patient care plan is the tool used to individualize patient care. Various forms may be used for documentation, and agency policy should be followed. Figure 4-3 shows a sample Nurses' Progress Notes. These notes reflect problem-oriented charting. Note how the specific nursing interventions and actions of the care plan are documented in the nurses' notes. Documentation of the care plan is essential and since the patient's care plan is individualized, it should be used as a guideline. The nurses' progress notes should indicate that the plan of care was followed.

The fourth step of the nursing process is implementation, putting the nursing interventions and actions into actual practice. The written care plan is used as a guide in administering patient care, in communicating with other members of the healthcare team, and in reporting patient

Figure 4-3 Nurses' Progress Notes

NURSES' PROGRESS NOTES

P—Problem, I—Intervention

Date	Hour	Remarks
4/2	0800	P # 1 Alterations in Bowel Elimination: Constipation Related to Immobility.
		I # 1 Fluids encouraged. Drank 150cc of warm water ac breakfast. Drank coffee and juice, total intake during breakfast 360cc. Intake recorded.
	0900	I # 1 Dietitian present, teaching patient re: fruit, bran, and food high in fiber. Drank water 200cc. Recorded on I & O record.
		Betty Scott, R.N.

information to the physician. While caring for your patient, you will note any changes, symptoms, or pertinent information. This should be reported to the nurse in charge so that the patient's care plan can be updated and modified as needed. If you are involved in the acute care setting, you will use the care plan as a guide for giving patient care, charting, giving reports to the R.N. and other healthcare team members, and continuing the data collection process.

The L.P.N./L.V.N. in the long-term care setting, i.e., nursing home and extended care, may work as a charge nurse managing patient care under the supervision of the registered nurse. While providing care to the patient, you should continue to make observations and to chart on the nurses' notes using the patient's care plan as a guide. The nursing diagnosis will assist in determining the priority of problems. When reporting to the R.N. and other healthcare team members, discuss the specific interventions or nursing actions in the care plan. Any changes or modifications can be made as needed, and the patient's care plan can be updated on a daily basis or as necessary. Figure 4-4 shows a nursing care plan for a patient receiving an angiogram. Note the separation of pre-angiography and postangiography problems listed in the "Usual Problems" section. The Nurses' Progress Notes in Figure 4-5 show the problem-oriented charting utilizing the care plan in Figure 4-4. Note the charting of specific interventions and the evaluation of observations and patient response.

Evaluation

Step 5 is evaluation. This final step includes looking at the nursing interventions to see how effective they have been. In other words, what you are evaluating is the patient's response to the care given. Evaluation of the care plan is a continous process, beginning as soon as nursing care is implemented. As discussed previously, data about the patient is collected continuously as the nursing care is given. This data collection and discussion of the nursing actions and interventions help make daily evaluation of the care plan an ongoing process.

Another important aspect of evaluation is determining if the goals/outcomes have been met. If they have not, perhaps the goals/outcomes need to be modified. Information for evaluation is obtained from the patient's responses to care given, ongoing patient observation, the patient's medical record, and members of the healthcare team. The care plan is centered on the patient, so the patient should be an active participant in evaluating care when possible. Often evaluation will show the need to reevaluate the patient's needs, the nursing diagnosis and interventions, and the patient care plan.

Figure 4–4 Angiogram Care Plan

USUAL PROBLEMS	EXPECTED OUTCOMES	DEADLINES	NURSING ORDERS
PREANGIOGRAPHY			
1. Fear due to unfamiliar procedure and unknown findings.	1. Verbalizes "I know what to expect during procedure." Relaxed appearance.	day of admission √ q 8 hr	1. Assign one R.N. to explain procedure, listen and reassure as needed. Prepare patient to expect: —Local anesthetic. —Medication to relax, but he will remain awake. —Small tube to be passed into artery through which dye containing iodine is injected. Dye enables blood vessels to be visible in X rays. —Certain discomforts during procedure: hard X-ray table for several hours, need to lie still, blushing, and brief pain in certain areas when dye is injected. —Bedrest for 6 hr post procedure. —Allow patient time to read "angiography

continued

51

Figure 4–4 *(Continued)*

USUAL PROBLEMS	EXPECTED OUTCOMES	DEADLINES	NURSING ORDERS
			explanation" on consent form before requesting signature.
2. Potential complications during or after procedure due to undetected physical abnormalities.	2. Prevention of avoidable complications by early detection of any abnormalities present before procedure.	day of admission ↓ q 8 hr	2A. On admission, ascertain if: —Allergic to iodine —Any history of bleeding tendencies B. On admission and q shift: —Palpate for presence or absence, strength vs. weakness of pulses. —Record vital signs and neurological signs.
POSTANGIOGRAPHY 1. Potential bleeding from puncture site.	1. No bleeding. Vital signs stable for patient.	After 6 hr ↓ q 2 hr	1A. Check puncture site for bleeding when taking vital signs. B. Maintain intact pressure dressing. C. Maintain complete bed rest for 6 hours post procedure or post bleeding.
2. Potential thrombus and/or neurological complications.	2. No sudden severe chest pain Pulse no weaker than before Vital signs and neurological signs within normal limits No seizures	After 24 hr ↓ q 8 hr	2. Check and record neurological signs when taking ordered vital signs.

Figure 4–5 Nurses' Progress Notes

P—Problem, I—Intervention

NURSES' PROGRESS NOTES (ANGIOGRAM)

Date	Hour	Remarks
4/1	0800	P # 1 Knowledge deficit related to angiogram.
		I # 1 Discussed with patient. Explained procedure for angiogram. Consent for angiogram
		obtained. Patient verbalized basic understanding of angiogram procedure.
	0930	I # 1 Reinforced explanation for purpose of medications prior to angiogram.
		Preangiogram medicines given as ordered.
Post	Angio	P # 1 Potential for hemorrhage from site of angiogram.
	1130	I#1 Vital signs monitored frequently, q 15 min times ½ hour.
		Pedal pulses checked, present 3 + bilaterally. Pressure dressing in place at site.
		Bedrest maintained. No evidence of bleeding, dressing dry and intact.
	1145	I#1 Vital signs stable, bedrest maintained, no evidence of bleeding, dressing
		dry and intact, pedal pulses 3 + bilaterally.
	1200	I#1 Bedrest maintained, vital signs stable, condition unchanged, no bleeding from
		site, pulses 3 + bilaterally, patient denies any discomfort.
		Mary Smith, R.N.

THE HEALTHCARE TEAM

The purposes of the healthcare agency are to provide care for the ill and injured, prevent disease, promote health, provide facilities for health education, and promote research in the sciences of medicine and nursing. The sophistication of technology and educational advancements require the skills and expertise of many people to carry out the purposes of healthcare institutions. The healthcare team includes everyone in the various departments associated with healthcare delivery. Each member of the healthcare team brings special expertise and skill to improve the quality of patient care.

The purpose of the team is to plan and coordinate the delivery of healthcare for the patient. Each member will have a different role or function, depending upon the needs of the patient and the specific problem identified. The team should be well organized and motivated by a mutual respect for the expertise and contribution of each team member. No one member is more important than the other. Some team members may have more contact with the patient than others, based on the patient needs.

Healthcare institutions vary in size depending on the services offered, number of personnel employed, and the size of the community served. Whatever the size, the institution is organized in a specific way. The departments may include administration, medical, nursing, therapy, laboratory, dietary, social services, medical records, auxilliary services, engineering, and radiology.

The various healthcare services provided can usually be found in one of the departments listed above. For example, therapy may include speech, occupational, physical, and respiratory therapies. Frequently, these professionals are included in the rehabilitation therapy department. The laboratory area may include histology, blood bank, microbiology, and medical technology. It is usually administered by a physician specialist, a pathologist. In larger instutitions, the blood bank may be managed under a separate department.

Adminstration is one of the largest departments in the healthcare institution. Its areas may include medical records, business/finance, personnel, public relations, community service, purchasing, and inpatient and outpatient admitting. Physicians, nurses, dietitians, and pharmacists are involved with the patient on a consistent twenty-four-hour basis. The physician is responsible for diagnosis and prescribed medical treatment. The dietitian focuses on the nutritional needs of the patient and works closely with the physicians and nurses. Usually, patients will require medications; the pharmacists are responsible for dispensing medications to the nursing units for patient administration. Nurses are in constant contact with patients and are responsible for a

Figure 4–6 Hospital Organizational Chart

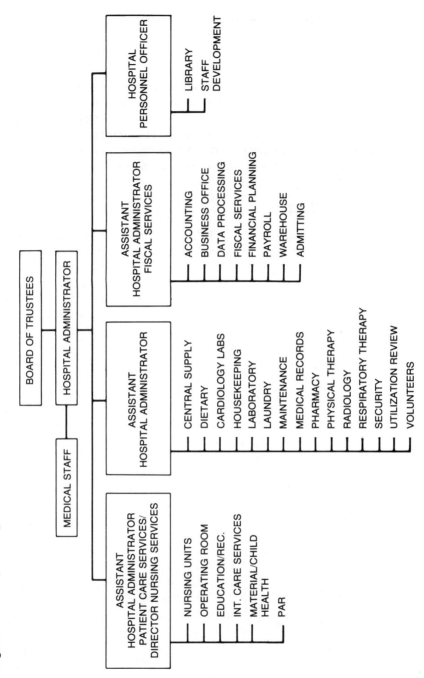

BOARD OF TRUSTEES

MEDICAL STAFF

HOSPITAL ADMINISTRATOR

ASSISTANT HOSPITAL ADMINISTRATOR PATIENT CARE SERVICES/ DIRECTOR NURSING SERVICES
- NURSING UNITS
- OPERATING ROOM
- EDUCATION/REC.
- INT. CARE SERVICES
- MATERIAL/CHILD HEALTH
- PAR

ASSISTANT HOSPITAL ADMINISTRATOR
- CENTRAL SUPPLY
- DIETARY
- CARDIOLOGY LABS
- HOUSEKEEPING
- LABORATORY
- LAUNDRY
- MAINTENANCE
- MEDICAL RECORDS
- PHARMACY
- PHYSICAL THERAPY
- RADIOLOGY
- RESPIRATORY THERAPY
- SECURITY
- UTILIZATION REVIEW
- VOLUNTEERS

ASSISTANT HOSPITAL ADMINISTRATOR FISCAL SERVICES
- ACCOUNTING
- BUSINESS OFFICE
- DATA PROCESSING
- FISCAL SERVICES
- FINANCIAL PLANNING
- PAYROLL
- WAREHOUSE
- ADMITTING

HOSPITAL PERSONNEL OFFICER
- LIBRARY
- STAFF DEVELOPMENT

significant portion of the patient care coordination and for nursing service delivery.

Ancillary personnel provide various healthcare services for the patient, some of which were previously handled by the professional workers. Because of the addition of various specialized health occupations, there has been an increase in the types of ancillary personnel. Nursing assistants, nursing technicians, pharmacy technicians, and ward clerks/unit secretaries are a part of the ancillary service personnel.

THE NURSING TEAM

The size and organization of the nursing team varies with each institution. Factors influencing the size and organization include bed capacity and the number of patients served, types of services offered, the complexity of the care needed, and the management philosophy of the institution's administration. Members of the nursing team include registered nurses, licensed practical/vocational nurses, student nurses, nursing assistants, and ward/unit clerks.

Each nursing department is organized differently. As a student nurse or a licensed nurse, it is your responsibility to know how your nursing department is organized. An example of an organizational chart for a nursing department appears on page 57. The organizational chart shows the lines of authority and responsibility. All nursing department personnel and students should work within those established lines of authority.

The person responsible for the delivery of nursing care may be called the director of nursing, nursing director, or assistant administrator for nursing. Some larger institutions use the title assistant administrator for nursing because the responsibilities are equal to those of an assistant administrator. Nursing is one of the largest departments in the facility both in care given and personnel employed, and the nursing department has twenty-four-hour contact with the patient, seven days a week.

Unit supervisors/clinical coordinators are responsible for various programs in the nursing area and report directly to the nursing administrator. Their responsibilities are to manage the patient care area(s) assigned, including staffing and the unit budget. The charge/head nurse is responsible for supervising care in the nursing area assigned and reports to the unit supervisor/clinical coordinator. In some facilities, the charge/head nurse is responsible for staff scheduling, with final approval given by the supervisor/clinical coordinator.

The Registered Nurse

Registered nurses are responsible for giving patient care and formulating a nursing diagnosis and a plan of care for each patient assigned. They

Figure 4–7 Nursing Department Organizational Chart

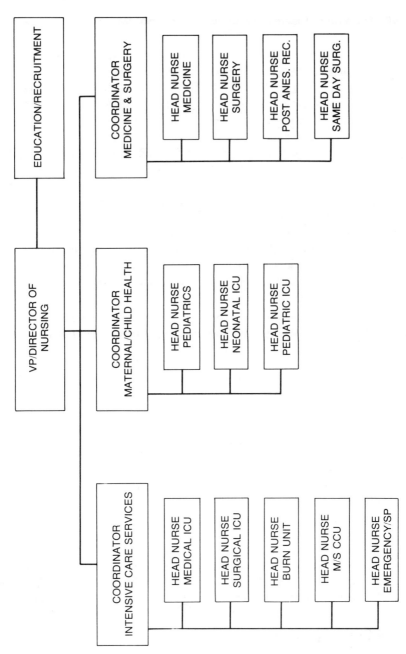

report directly to the team leader or to the charge/head nurse, depending on the organization of the nursing department. Staff nurses plan nursing care to be delivered and work closely with other hospital personnel to provide patient care and services. The registered nurse works independently when performing nursing activities and dependently when carrying out the prescribed orders of the physician.

The educational programs for the professional nurse are two-, three-, and four-year programs. The two-year program includes general education courses, nursing theory, and clinical experience. Graduates receive an associate's degree upon completion. A graduate of the three-year program receives a diploma; the courses include general education and nursing theory courses, and emphasis is placed on clinical experience. The four-year graduate receives a baccalaureate degree in nursing; the course work includes nursing theory and the arts and sciences. The graduates of all the programs are eligible to take the R.N. licensing examination in their individual states.

The Licensed Practical/Vocational Nurse

Practical/vocational nurses provide bedside patient care under the supervision of the registered nurse, physician, or dentist. While providing direct patient care, the practical nurse is in a strategic position to observe the patient's response to treatment and care. As an effective and contributing member of the nursing team, the practical/vocational nurse assists in implementation of the patient's care plan.

In long-term and intermediate care facilities, the practical nurse may be responsible for supervising nursing care delivery to a group of patients. In this setting, the practical nurse may administer medications and treatments to the patients assigned, while supervising nursing assistants in the performance of basic nursing functions such as bathing and hygiene care.

The educational course for the practical/vocational nurse is usually one year in length. Course offerings include nursing theory, biological sciences, and clinical experience. Graduates of these programs are issued a certificate or diploma and are eligible to take the licensing examination.

The Student Nurse

The student nurse is an active member of the nursing team and works under the direct supervision of the clinical nursing instructor. The clinical experience is an extension of the classroom learning experience. Students are expected to provide safe and appropriate care to the patients assigned and to assist other members of the team. The clinical area provides an opportunity for the student to apply what has been learned in the classroom. While the student nurse is a part of the nursing team, students do not replace staff and should not be included as staff in the various staffing reports and records. Because students are expected to provide safe and responsible patient care, the clinical instructor is legally responsible for student activities. The clinical instructor and students work closely in a team effort with supervisors, head nurses, and other members of the nursing and healthcare teams.

The Nursing Assistant

Nursing assistants assist in providing basic nursing care to patients. They work under the direct supervision of the registered nurse or the licensed practical/vocational nurse. Their duties can include bathing and feeding patients, serving trays and providing fresh water, taking vital signs, making beds, ambulating patients, and serving nourishments.

Nursing assistants are valuable, contributing members of the nursing care team due to their direct and continuous association with the patient. Their assistance in observing the patient and reporting accurately to the nurse contributes to the success of the nursing team.

Education for the nursing assistant is provided in vocational/technical schools and in on the job programs. The on-the-job programs are sometimes located in healthcare institutions; the classroom instruction and clinical supervision are provided by registered nurses and practical/vocational nurses. The programs in vocational/technical schools include classroom instruction and clinical experience. A local hospital or long-term-care agency offers their facility to provide the clinical experience. Both types of programs range from six weeks to three months in length. Graduates receive a certificate, some states require an examination for certification.

The Ward/Unit Clerk

The ward/unit clerk is responsible primarily for the secretarial duties for the patient care area. These duties include completing reports and records under supervision, completing requisitions for patient tests and treatments, initiating papers for patient discharges and transfers, scheduling appointments for various patient services, answering the telephone, routing reports and records to other departments, recording information from the chart to the kardex or other records, ordering supplies and maintaining inventories, setting up charts for new admissions, distributing the mail, receiving and forwarding messages, and keeping supply shelves stocked.

Educational preparation includes on-the-job training and training in technical schools. Training usually takes three to six months, and graduates receive a certificate upon completion.

NURSING SERVICE DELIVERY

There are four popular methods of delivering nursing care: the case method, functional nursing, team nursing, and primary care nursing. The goal of any method of nursing care delivery is to give the optimum care in the most efficient manner with the least cost. Each institution has a different method of delivery of nursing care. Several factors must be considered in determining the system of choice, such as the physical size of the hospital, the variety of services offered, appropriate staff with required skills levels, the type of equipment available, and the availability of appropriate contract services.

Case Nursing   *case management*

In this method of delivering nursing care, one nurse is responsible for the total care of one or more patients for one shift. This method has been used since the early 1920s and is the oldest approach to nursing care delivery. It is also called comprehensive care or total care nursing. It is used in private-duty nursing and in intensive care and special-care units. Instructors frequently use this method when making patient assignments for student nurses.

Functional Nursing

This method of organizing nursing care delivery is based on task orientation. The nursing care for a specific group of patients is divided into the tasks necessary for patient care. Each member of the nursing team is assigned a function or task according to individual skills and abilities. For example, one person may be assigned all the vital signs, another team member may be the medication nurse, and another team member may make the beds.

Functional nursing is efficient because fewer team members are required to carry out the tasks, and each staff member is utilized to the fullest extent. However, patients get fragmented care because many staff members are responsible for many functions, and patients often complain that they are not sure who is responsible for their care. Establishing patient rapport is frequently a difficult task.

Team Nursing

Team nursing was introduced during the 1950s. In this method, a team of staff members is responsible for the care of a group of patients. Each team member cares for a certain number of patients, and the patient assignments are based on the needs of the patients and the skills of the team members. The team's activities are coordinated by a team leader, usually a registered nurse. The team leader is also responsible for planning and evaluating the care given in addition to supervising the personnel in the team. Each member's contribution is considered important, and the abilities of each team member are used effectively.

An important part of team nursing is the patient care conference, held daily and attended by all team members. During the conference, patient information is discussed among the members, and patient care plans are updated and modified as needed.

Primary Care Nursing

This method was developed in 1968 and is used by many hospitals today. In primary care nursing, a registered nurse has responsibility for a patient for twenty-four hours a day until the patient is discharged or transferred. The primary nurse is responsible for the admission assessment and interview, develops the nursing care plan, and evaluates the care given. The primary nurse works with two other nurses who are responsible for the patient during the two shifts when the primary care nurse is not present. The two associate nurses are responsible to the primary care nurse and use the nursing care plan as a basis for their nursing actions. The associate nurse may be a registered nurse or a licensed practical/ vocational nurse.

Some hospitals have found that primary care nursing improves the continuity of patient care. Others have found this method too costly because of the number of registered nurses required.

REVIEW/DISCUSSION/ACTIVITIES _____

1. List the skills required to manage activities relative to time.
2. Identify a time waster in your life. Develop a plan toward a solution and discuss in a class discussion group.
3. Review the section on taking notes during a lecture and discuss those techniques you find helpful.
4. Develop a study schedule. What personal adjustments were necessary in developing this study schedule?

BIBLIOGRAPHY _____

Carpenito, L.J. *Nursing Diagnosis: Application to Clinical Practice.* Philadelphia: J.B. Lippincott, 1983.

Ellis, J.R., and Hartley, C.L. *Nursing in Today's World: Challenges, Issues and Trends.* Philadelphia: J.B. Lippincott, 1988.

Hand, Lee. *Nursing Supervision.* Reston, Va.: Prentice-Hall, 1981.

Henderson, V. *The Nature of Nursing: A Definition and Its Implication for* Practice, Research and Education. New York: Macmillan, 1966.

CHAPTER
5

Healthcare Delivery System/Healthcare Agencies

OBJECTIVES

The student successfully attaining the goals of this chapter will be able to:

- Describe official and voluntary public health agencies.
- Provide examples of private and public healthcare agencies.
- Give examples of intermediate and intensive care units in hospitals.
- Describe preventive, primary, secondary, tertiary, and continuing care.
- Describe two types of health insurance.

The healthcare system includes healthcare financing, healthcare regulation, healthcare providers, and healthcare services. As a student, you are a member of the healthcare system. You are one of the many providers of healthcare. The purpose of healthcare agencies is to serve the healthcare needs of the public. A healthcare agency can provide for healthcare needs in several ways: patient education, education of healthcare workers, administration of patient care, and treatment research.

A healthcare provider may be an individual healthcare worker or an institution or group that provides healthcare services. Physicians, nurse practitioners, and podiatrists are examples of individual healthcare providers. Individual practitioners do refer patients to institutions that provide healthcare services. For example, a physician may send a patient to a particular hospital or clinic for surgery, treatment, or diagnostic tests. Health maintenance organizations are examples of group healthcare providers. Hospitals, outpatient clinics, nursing homes, and ambulatory services clinics are examples of institutional healthcare providers.

The care delivered by the various healthcare providers is considered a service. The service delivered is determined by the type of agency or individual provider. The service can be actual patient care, diagnostic tests, treatment, or a patient educational program on wellness aimed at the prevention of illness. Figure 5-1 lists the five basic functions and purposes of healthcare institutions.

Healthcare providers are certified, governed, licensed, and registered by various regulating agencies and associations. This regulation is necessary to protect the public receiving the services and to maintain the

FIVE BASIC FUNCTIONS AND PURPOSES OF HEALTH CARE INSTITUTIONS:

1 TO PROVIDE CARE FOR ILL AND/OR INJURED

2 TO PREVENT DISEASE

3 TO PROMOTE INDIVIDUAL AND COMMUNITY HEALTH

4 TO PROVIDE FACILITIES FOR THE EDUCATION OF HEALTH WORKERS

5 TO PROMOTE RESEARCH IN THE SCIENCES OF MEDICINE AND NURSING

Figure 5–1   Five Basic Functions and Purposes of Healthcare Institutions

quality of health care. Healthcare regulation and financing will be discussed in more detail later in this chapter.

HEALTHCARE DELIVERY SYSTEM

The healthcare delivery system is divided into two main service divisions or categories: public and private.

Public Health Organizations

There are two types of public health organizations: official and voluntary. Official healthcare agencies are set up by the federal, state, county, or city government and they are tax supported. The Department of Health and Human Services, established in 1980, is the health agency at the federal level. The U.S. Public Health Service is a division of the Department of Health and Human Services. Each state has a state health department; the health agency at the local level is the city or county health department. Official public healthcare organizations generally deliver services in the area of disease prevention and wellness promotion.

Hospitals owned by the local, state, or federal government are public hospitals. County hospitals are owned by the local government. A state mental hospital is an example of a state-owned hospital. Military hospitals and veterans hospitals are examples of federally owned hospitals.

Voluntary healthcare agencies are nonprofit agencies set up to serve the general public. They are supported by patient fees and voluntary donations. The agencies are administered by a board of directors or trustees. Voluntary agencies may offer health services to the patient, but, the primary focus is education and research. Examples of voluntary healthcare agencies include hospitals, American Lung Association, American Cancer Society, Visiting Nurse Associations, Alcoholics Anonymous, Al-Anon, and the Easter Seal Society.

Private Healthcare Agencies

Private healthcare agencies are privately owned and operated by an individual or a group of people. They are operated for profit and administered by the owners. The following discussion provides examples of private healthcare agencies.

Hospitals. They may be nonprofit or for profit. Private hospitals referred to as voluntary hospitals are operated by partnerships, corporations, or religious associations. These hospitals are considered not-for-profit or nonproprietary.. Hospitals operated for profit are called proprietary or for-profit hospitals.

Hospitals can be classified not only by ownership, but also by the bed capacity, the variety of services provided, and the patient length of stay. The bed capacity of hospitals can range from 20 to 1000 or even more and may provide both inpatient and outpatient services. Many large hospitals are associated with colleges and universities and offer teaching and medical research activities.

Hospitals providing care for acute and chronic conditions to patients of all ages are called general hospitals. Children's hospitals and orthopedic hospitals are examples of specialty hospitals because they offer care for specific conditions and illnesses.

Long-term hospitals provide care to patients needing extended care, i.e., for thirty days or more. Short-term hospital patients usually stay less than thirty days and receive care for short term acute conditions and illnesses.

The various patient units in a hospital are distinguished or separated by the type of care and service required by the patients. Some units are larger than others, depending on the complexity of care and the specialized personnel and equipment needed. Patients requiring general acute care for conditions and illnesses are grouped in medical-surgical units. The medical-surgical unit is considered an intermediate care unit because the patients are not critically ill, but they do require specialized acute care. The maternity unit, nursery, and the pediatric units are included in the intermediate care unit group.

Patients who are critically ill and require intensive specialized care are admitted to varying types of intensive care units. These units include medical/surgical intensive care unit, coronary care unit, pediatric intensive care unit, and the postanesthesia recovery unit.

Home Healthcare Agencies. Various services are offered, including nursing, homemaking, companion services, and physical and occupational therapies.

Extended Care. Extended Care Units (ECUs) are frequently associated with hospitals. These units provide nursing care for patients who require additional time to recover from an acute hospital stay before being discharged home.

Nursing Homes. Nursing homes provide various levels of care— skilled, intermediate, and custodial. Frequently, the majority of patients cared for in these agencies are the elderly and the terminally ill. Other types of patients include the homeless, the disabled, and the helpless. Quite often, the nursing home becomes the patient's home. The patient in the long-term-care setting is often referred to as "resident."

Ambulatory Surgery Facilities.   These surgery centers provide certain types of surgeries and permit the patient to be admitted early in the morning, have the surgical procedure, recover from anesthesia, receive necessary nursing care and treatment, and be discharged late afternoon or early evening of the same day. This eliminates the need for an overnight hospital stay and is less costly for the patient.

Ambulatory Care Agencies.   Patients can be seen for primary healthcare services on a walk-in basis. Usually patients do not need an appointment, and the service is fast. Some of these agencies have extended hours, which many people find convenient, and serve persons who may not have a family physician.

Ambulatory/Outpatient Clinics.   Outpatient ambulatory clinics provide care for patients who do not require hospitalization and for patients who need follow-up care after hospitalization. Frequently, these clinics are associated with acute hospitals, and patients are seen by appointment.

LEVELS OF HEALTH CARE

The healthcare delivery system includes several levels of care. The *level of care* refers to the complexity of the patient's needs, the level of skills needed by the personnel, and the equipment required for the care of the patient. Nurses are involved in all levels of health care delivery. The various levels include preventive, primary, secondary, tertiary, and continuing care.

Preventive Care

Preventive care is becoming more popular as the healthcare consumer becomes more knowledgeable about individual health needs. A focus on promoting wellness has resulted in a variety of services being offered in this area of health care. Practical/vocational nurses are involved in preventive care through community service agencies, health screening clinics, and public health agencies.

Primary Care

The focus of primary care is early detection and diagnosis and disease prevention. These services are provided by doctors and nurse practitioners in outpatient/ ambulatory care facilities, offices, and clinics.

Secondary Health Care

Secondary health care is administered at a hospital that has personnel, equipment, and services of a specialized nature. The care emphasis is on the diagnosis, treatment, care, and related services required by the patient. The patient's care and all services rendered are controlled and supervised by the patient's physician. At this level of care, the patient usually requires the services of specialized equipment and personnel on a consistent, around-the-clock basis.

Tertiary Care

The goal of tertiary care is to restore the patient to maximum functioning after an acute or chronic illness or trauma. Healthcare workers providing tertiary care need specialized education. Their patients usually have illnesses or injuries involving the musculoskeletal or neurological systems. Tertiary care can be provided in therapy centers, either free standing or associated with acute hospitals, in long-term-care facilities, or through home nursing agencies.

Continuing Care

Continuing care is provided on a long-term basis in facilities such as inpatient care centers for the disabled, nursing homes, hospice care centers, residential care homes, geriatric daycare centers, and personal care homes. Nurses are involved at this level to coordinate care, provide treatment, and administer medication.

FINANCING HEALTHCARE SERVICES

Health care is expensive, so expensive that many people cannot afford the cost of quality health care. The Department of Health and Human Services estimates that by the year 2000, more than $500 billion will be spent yearly for health care. A significant portion of healthcare costs is paid by private and government health insurance.

Private Medical Insurance

Private medical insurance can be purchased by a group or on an individual basis. The cost of the insurance varies with the type and amount of coverage desired. Some insurance plans pay only for those services specifically covered in the policy, and usually the subscriber may choose the care provider as long as exclusions do not exist.

In prepaid private insurances, the subscriber pays a set periodic charge, which permits the subscriber to use the plan's services. The cost of the plan is based on the services offered. A health maintenance organization, (HMO), is an example of prepaid insurance; subscribers must receive services by HMO provider members.

Government Medical Insurance

The Social Security Act of 1965 included provisions for a federally sponsored insurance plan. Title XVIII, Medicare, is the federal insurance plan; Title XIX, Medicaid, is a federal–state insurance plan.

Medicare provides health insurance for persons 65 years of age and older. Part A of Medicare insurance also provides hospital insurance to persons under sixty-five years of age who are permanently and totally disabled. Patients with end-stage kidney disease are also eligible for these benefits. Part B of Medicare includes inpatient/outpatient physician services and other services for persons over sixty-five years of age. There are eligibility requirements for both Part A and Part B. Part A is available without cost, but there is a deductible. Part B requires a monthly premium. Medicare insurance is funded through Social Security taxes paid to the federal government.

Medicaid insurance pays for healthcare services for low income families and the poor who are unable to obtain private insurance coverage because of the costs involved. Medicaid is paid for through federal and state funds.

Diagnosis-Related Groups

In 1983, in an effort to reduce the rising cost of health care associated with the Medicare program, the Health Care Financing Administration adopted a prospective payment method. In this system, rates and fees for healthcare services are set in advance, so hospitals know how much they will be reimbursed before services are provided.

The diagnosis-related groups (DRGs) are used for grouping or classifying patients based on medical diagnosis. Patients are placed in a DRG based on diagnosis and age, and each diagnosis-related group has a specified amount of money that will be paid by Medicare.

The prospective payment method system provides for care of the patient and includes a profit for the hospital. When the patient receives care and is discharged within the guidelines of the DRGs, the difference in cost is retained by the hospital; however, if the patient stays in the hospital longer than the Medicare insurance will pay, then the hospital has to make up the difference in costs. When healthcare providers are aware of the prospective payment system for Medicare patients, healthcare services can be rendered with controlled costs.

HEALTH CARE REGULATION

Hospitals and nursing homes must be approved by their state department of health. There is a periodic evaluation process, and the facility must meet certain criteria to receive approval to operate in that state. Many hospitals and nursing homes receive accreditation from the American Hospital Association. The accreditation process is voluntary; when accreditation is received, it means that the hospital or nursing home surpasses the minimum standards of approval for facility operation. The Joint Commission on Accreditation of Hospitals (JCAH), is an organization with member representation from the American College of Physicians, American College of Surgeons, Americam Medical Association, and the American Hospital Association. The process utililized is an evaluation based on specific standards and criteria, and again participation in the process is voluntary. When the requirements are met, hospitals receive accreditation for a specified period of time. Hospitals must be accredited to receive Medicare funds, to sponsor internships and residency programs, and to be eligible for many of the insurance plans that operate nationally.

The Department of Health and Human Services regulations require hospitals to establish various review committees. One of the functions of these committees is to review the medical care provided to patients whose hospitalization is paid for by Medicare, Medicaid, and Maternal and Child Health Insurance. Additional duties include the study and review of the utilization of hospital facilities.

The American Medical Association has developed a Peer Review Manual, which provides guidelines for committee development, review concepts, and program implementation. Peer review focuses on review of professional practice of individual practitioners by practicing members of the same profession.

Nursing participates in this quality review process by conducting and participating in nursing audits. A nurse peer group will conduct concurrent and retrospective review of care for the purpose of quality assurance. Concurrent review is an examination of the patient's progress while patient care and treatment are still in progress. Retrospective review examines past or completed work with patients and their treatment and care. Documentation in the patient's medical record is the source of information for the review. In the concurrent review process, documentation of care in the patient's medical record is used, along with interview, observation, and inspection of the patient. Concurrent review has the advantage of providing an opportunity to make changes in ongoing care.

Physicians, nurse practitioners, dentists, and podiatrists are considered primary healthcare providers and must be licensed by the state in which they practice. As a nurse, you will be required to be licensed in order to work as a practical/vocational nurse. Licensure of practitioners protects the public consumer. Licensing agencies or boards are responsible for issuing licenses after successful completion of licensure examination requirements. Their duties also include renewal, suspension, and revoking of licenses. Other board/agency functions are discussed later in the text.

REVIEW/DISCUSSION/ACTIVITIES

1. What are the five basic functions and purposes of healthcare institutions? Give examples of each.
2. List the levels of health care and discuss examples of each.
3. Research one of the health care regulatory agencies and discuss in class.

BIBLIOGRAPHY

Dugas, B. *Introduction to Patient Care: A Comprehensive Approach to Nursing.* 4th ed. Philadelphia: W.B. Saunders, 1983.

Hawkins, J. W., Hayes, E.R., and Abner, C.S.: *An Orientation to Hospitals and Community Agencies.* New York: Springer Verlag, 1986.

Hill, S.S., and Howlett, H.A.: *Success in Practical Nursing: Personal and Vocational Issues.* Philadelphia: W.B. Saunders, 1988.

Roemer, M.I.: *An Introduction to the U.S. Health Care System.* New York: Springer Verlag, 1986.

Rowland, H.S., and Rowland, B.L.: *Nursing Administration Handbook.* Germantown, MD: Aspen, 1980.

Williams, S., and Torrens, P. *Introduction to Health Services.* New York: Wiley, 1980.

Wolff, L. *Fundamentals of Nursing,* 7th ed. Philadelphia: J.B. Lippincott, 1983.

CHAPTER

6

The Patient

OBJECTIVES

The student successfully attaining the goals of this chapter will be able to:

- Define culture, and explain the importance of the nurse's awareness of cultural differences when giving patient care.
- Identify areas in which patients may differ culturally.
- Describe four types of communication.
- Identify six ways to promote effective communication.
- Identify at least five barriers to effective communication.
- Describe the importance of empathy in the nurse–patient relationship.

Nurses use specialized skills to care for people who are sick. All persons have basic human needs, and these basic needs are used as a basis for planning patient care. Each patient you encounter is different from other patients. In many instances, your patients will be different from you in values, personal beliefs, life styles, personal approach, and in a variety of other ways. It is important to remember to refrain in making judgments about people who are different from you. A part of your responsibility as a nurse is to accept and respect the human individuality of patients. This does not mean that you personally accept the differences or that you offer approval, but all patients deserve and expect quality nursing care.

Your patients may act and think differently than you because of personal beliefs and value systems, ethnic background, economic status, religion, educational preparation, and many other factors. As a nurse, you must continue to respect the human individuality of your patients and consistently provide quality nursing care.

CULTURAL AND ETHNIC DIVERSITIES

Culture is learned behavior and consists of all of the beliefs, values, attitudes, ideas, and methods of doing things employed by a group of people. Customs are important to individual cultures because they signify the shared and accepted ways of doing things by the people of a particular culture. *Ethnic* is a term applied to various groups of people who share racial, language, historical, and religious similarities and customs.

Cultural and ethnic differences are a part of a person's personality and are visible in human interaction and behaviors. As a nurse, it is your responsibility to develop an appreciation and an awareness of cultural and ethnic differences when taking care of your patients. By understanding the differences, you can avoid assumptions, confusion, and misunderstandings. When learning about various cultural and ethnic groups, it is important to remember to use the information as a guideline. The information obtained may describe a group of people in general terms, but not the individuals in the group. For example, it is a false assumption that all people with a Mexican heritage eat or enjoy spicy foods.

Areas that may differ culturally include communication or language, religion, educational preparation, and economic status.

When your patient speaks a different language, this can be a barrier that limits communication and understanding. This is frustrating for the patient and for the nurse, and it can be potentially unsafe for the patient if there is a delay in patient care. This situation can create a sense of isolation and fear for the patient, seriously hampering patient care. Most hospitals publish a list of hospital staff members who are fluent in various languages or of persons outside the hospital who volunteer their services as interpreters. This list includes the person's name, the department of employment, the telephone number, and the hours of availability. It is an important list and is usually included as a part of the nursing orientation for new employees.

Communication will be discussed later in this chapter under "Nurse–Patient Communication."

Religion is very personal and fundamental to those who have religious beliefs. Spiritual fulfillment provides meaning and purpose to life for some, and for others is a source of strength and hope. Many of your patients will be dealing with issues of health, life, or death and may turn to their religion as a source of comfort.

Many hospitals have pastoral care departments with members of the clergy, nuns, and layperson volunteers. You may be asked to call a member of this department to provide assistance to your patient or to the patient's family. Some hospitals have a social services department; a part of their responsibility is to call various community religious volunteers to come in and provide spiritual care. In many hospitals, the patients are visited by a religious volunteer, layperson, or clergy member on a daily or periodic basis. As a nurse, you will be asked to accommodate patient religious beliefs and practices whenever possible.

Some hospitals have chapels where patients and families may go for worship services or meditation. You can provide information to the patient and family regarding the availability of the chaplain, the chapel, or religious services at the hospital.

There may be situations in which a patient's religious beliefs interfere with medical treatment and nursing care. For example, some patients may not be able to eat certain foods based on their religion, or they may not be able to receive specialized medical treatment. A patient belonging to the Jehovah's Witnesses is not permitted to receive blood transfusions. In these situations, the nurse can consult with the clergy for possible resolutions, but the patient does have the right to refuse treatment and care.

The educational preparation and economic level of your patients are often closely associated. These two areas should be taken into consideration when you are doing patient teaching. Avoid using language that is above or below your patient's level of understanding. In either case, it can be insulting or demeaning to the patient. It is important to tailor your teaching and explanations to the patient's level of understanding.

The patient's economic level will determine their ability to pay for certain services and medications and the availability to them of certain special foods. This can be especially important to patients being discharged from the hospital who require certain specialized services from various providers and healthcare agencies. Patients on therapeutic or special diets may find that they are unable to purchase foods required because of the costs involved. As a nurse, you become a resource person for your patient. You should be aware of the various local community healthcare services available and how to access them. Additionally, as a healthcare practitioner, you become a referral-resource person for your patient.

NURSE–PATIENT RELATIONSHIPS _____

Today's relationship between nurse and patient has changed as dramatically as the times have changed. The healthcare consumer is a product of the information age. The level of education of the public has increased, and people are more knowledgeable about health, wellness, and illness than ever before. As a result, today's patients are actively participating in their care. They expect to be actively involved and informed about decisions affecting their health and well-being.

Nursing involves encouraging and supporting active participation of the patient in problem identification and in the nursing care plan. The patient today takes a more collaborative role, and the nurse–patient therapeutic relationship is best characterized as a partnership.

An effective nurse–patient relationship ideally is characterized by trust and confidence in the nurse; a feeling of independence and appropriate participation of the patient; continuity and flexibility of the relationship; and reasonable expectations on the part of both nurse and patient.

As a student nurse, you will acquire the essential elements to help you become an effective and contributing member of the healthcare team. At the same time, you will be experiencing personal growth, becoming more aware of who you are as a person, and becoming more accepting of self. This personal growth leads to self-confidence. Self-confidence and sound educational preparation will prepare you to be secure in developing nurse–patient relationships. Patients appreciate a nurse who is self-confident and knowledgeable and shows respect and concern for their well-being.

Initial trust in the nurse's skill is usually created by the degree of confidence the nurse communicates through personal style and manner. Trust and confidence are built when the nurse provides support, yet respects the patient's independence. Trust and confidence are also created when a reserve is maintained that defines the nurse as a person whose aim is to help.

The mutual participation relationship is most desirable because the patient feels some responsibility for a successful outcome, which involves both active participation and a feeling of personal responsibility for one's behavior. This is created by appropriate use of the nurse's authority. Some dependence on the nurse is useful and appropriate, especially in acute and frightening illnesses and conditions, but it is generally not useful to foster the patient's feeling of dependence. Dependence can interfere with patient treatment and care. The best nurse–patient relationship encourages the patient to take increasing self responsibility, at a time and rate consistent with good treatment and care.

The nurse–patient relationship has continuity and flexibility. It is a continuing relationship because the nurse has consistent contact with the patient during the hospital stay. There are times when the relationship is more intense and involves more frequent contact with the patient. For example, during the immediate, acute, postoperative phase of a patient's hospital stay, the patient requires intense care and treatment. Other times, the nurse may make frequent short visits with the patient. An example of an appropriate short visit would be on the third or fourth postoperative day if the patient is progressing well—the need for intensive care is diminished and, consequently, it is not necessary for the nurse to continue to provide an intensive level of care. The nature and severity of the patient's condition influences the level of the nurse's involvement.

The relationship between nurse and patient begins when the patient is admitted to the patient care unit. The nurse interviews the patient to obtain information about health problems and issues. This information is used to formulate the patient care plan. To make the patient feel more at ease, the nurse should provide some orientation to the room and to the unit. To ensure that the nurse–patient relationship begins in a positive direction, the nurse must demonstrate competence, listening skills, courtesy and respect, and effective communication skills and techniques.

During the working phase of the nurse–patient relationship, both patient and nurse make decisions about the patient's care and set about to put the care plan in action. When the patient's condition improves or changes and warrants a different level of care, the nurse–patient relationship also changes. Preparing the patient for discharge involves teaching and giving instructions regarding care, follow-up appointments, and various services available in the community. This is the terminating phase of the relationship and is generally a mutually satisfying experience for both nurse and patient.

NURSE–PATIENT COMMUNICATION _____

Communication is an exchange of information, it is a continuous process that occurs with every patient contact. Comunication can occur through touch, silence, verbally, or nonverbally.

Touch is a form of nonverbal communication that can relay different messages to different people, and so should be used with care and judgment. Nurses are in close physical contact when giving care to patients, so touch is a part of nursing. Usually, the touch carries the message of caring, but some people do not like to be touched, and the nurse must always respect the patient's feelings.

Effective communication includes silence. Silence is appropriate when your patient may want to reflect on a life experience. A hospice patient once requested that a nurse "just sit with me for a few minutes." Silence can be an expression of comfort. Other times, your patient may be having some fears and apprehension about tests and procedures, but may be too afraid to discuss them. When the nurse recognizes this fear, an explanation about tests and procedures can be reassuring. Many times, however, the importance of silence in communication can be overlooked.

Verbal communication uses words and includes speaking, reading, and writing. When working with your patients, be alert to observe nonverbal communication carefully while you listen to what your patient is saying. There are many things that can be done to promote effective communication with patients; the following are a few suggestions.

1. Keep your mind open. Do not prejudge your patient, which blocks communication because you may not receive the correct message or the message intended.
2. Have some knowledge of the subject you discuss with the patient; if you do not know something admit so and make an offer to obtain the information. The patient will quickly realize if you are not knowledgeable about a topic and may lose confidence in you as a caregiver and resource person.
3. Focus the conversation on the patient and show interest in what the patient is saying. The conversation should not be focused on the caregiver. You can show interest and attention by using eye-to-eye contact, by sitting down when convenient, and by listening attentively when the patient is talking.
4. Provide privacy and let the patient know that conversations will be kept in confidence. Patients will not be comfortable in discussing issues with you if they feel that the conversation will be overheard by others. Confidentiality is important to the patient, but you must tell your patient that you will have to share information with appropriate healthcare team members if you believe the information will affect the treatment and care.
5. Use language the patient understands. Communication is lost if you use language the patient cannot understand. Patients have a right to make their own decisions and necessary information should be pro-

vided. Do not give advice unless advice is requested. Even if advice is requested, follow your hospital's policy or contact your unit supervisor for correct procedure to follow. In all cases, be very accurate when providing information.

6. Continue to observe your patient with appropriate use of touch and silence and have a purpose for conversation. The patient may exhibit some important gestures or nonverbal signs that may more accurately describe their feelings. Sometimes what is said does not reflect the exact feeling one may be experiencing. Always have a purpose for conversation so that idle "chit-chat" does not become the main subject or the primary reason for the conversation. This will also help both you and the patient to stay focused on the subject.

During nonverbal communication, information is exchanged without using words through posture, gestures, facial expressions, sounds such as crying or laughing, general physical appearance, dress, and grooming. Frequently, it is easy to see certain feelings your patient might be experiencing, such as happiness, pain, and sadness through laughter, facial grimacing, or crying. Depression and feelings of poor self-worth are often noticed in one's personal grooming, dress, and physical appearance. Communication experts say that the nonverbal communications are more difficult to control, and feelings and messages are often communicated more accurately through nonverbal communication.

BARRIERS TO EFFECTIVE NURSE–PATIENT COMMUNICATION

Several approaches have been identified as barriers to effective communication and should be avoided by the nurse when communicating with patients. Responses and statements that do not promote effective communication and nurse–patient relationships may include the following.

1. Stereotyped responses may leave the impression that the nurse is not listening or that an answer has been prepared in advance. The patient may believe that their concerns are not important enough to receive your full attention. An example of a stereotyped statement by a nurse is "Everybody is scared of that procedure" or "Nobody likes hospital food."

2. "You will do just fine" and "Everything is going to be great" are examples of pat answers. As with stereotyped responses, pat answers can convey a lack of interest or minimize the importance of individual feelings and concerns.

3. Lecturing the patient does not promote an environment for developing effective nurse–patient relationships. This can be demeaning and belittles the patient and is an inappropriate emphasis of the nurse's authority and knowledge.
4. Probing can be interpreted as an invasion of privacy and may cause patients to avoid conversation. Always explain the purpose of the conversation and tell the patient why you need the information. When you are seeking information, do not ask closed questions that require a yes or no answer. Ask questions that require the patient to provide an explanation, such as "Tell me about your pain" or "What side effects are you experiencing from taking this medication?"

Other approaches that should be avoided include, threatening the patient, shaming and criticizing, providing unwanted and unrequested advice, and offering unrealistic assurance and hope.

COMMUNICATING EMPATHY/EMOTIONAL SUPPORT _____

The patient's emotional state will be affected by actual or potential physical illness. This can be expressed through some common emotional reactions. Patients may experience these reactions in varying degrees depending on past experiences related to illness, the severity of the health issue, whether or not other problems are involved, and individual personal style.

As a nurse, you are in a position to provide support, understanding, and encouragement to your patients. Empathy is the ability to understand what the other person is feeling, without experiencing it yourself. Empathy demonstrates caring and support. However, it will not be possible to empathize with all of your patients because of limited personal experience with illness and various treatments and care.

Empathy permits the patient to experience the illness or condition with the knowledge that the nurse understands the situation and is there to provide support and encouragement. it allows the nurse to maintain the reserve and distance necessary to remain objective and provide the care needed, while showing a caring and supportive concern for the patient.

Because physical and emotional energies are among your assets, you must avoid draining yourself by becoming too closely involved with the situation. This prevents you from helping the patient because you will no longer be able to maintain the objectivity required in caring for the patient and in making appropriate decisions.

REVIEW/DISCUSSION/ACTIVITIES

1. Discuss the cultural differences existing in the local communities that can have a significant impact in patient care situations.
2. Identify hospital services that provide assistance to patients and families of ethnic and cultural differences.
3. Identify and discuss the impact of patient cultural differences on the therapeutic nurse–patient relationship. Provide examples.
4. List and discuss suggestions to promote effective communication with patients.

BIBLIOGRAPHY

Brownlee, A. *Community, Culture and Care: A Cross Cultural Guide for Health Workers*. St. Louis: C.V. Mosby, 1978.

Burnard, P. "Learning to Communicate." *Nursing Mirror* 161 (1985): 30–31.

Gerrard, B; Boniface, W.; and Love, B. *Interpersonal Skills for Health Professionals*. East Norwalk, Ct.: Appleton & Lange, 1980.

Keane, C. B. *Essentials of Medical-Surgical Nursing*. Philadelphia: W.B. Saunders, 1986.

Milliken, M. *Understanding Human Behavior: A Guide for Health Care Workers,* 3d ed. Albany, N.Y.: Delmar Publishers, 1981.

Thompson, R. L. "Communicator's Checklist." *Caring* 3 (1984): 32–38, 40.

CHAPTER

7

Legal Awareness

OBJECTIVES

The student successfully attaining the goals of this chapter will be able to:

- Define common law and statutory law.
- Explain the purposes of the medical chart.
- Explain the various legal documents as presented.
- List reasons for patient litigations as presented.
- Identify factors that reduce the risk of lawsuits.
- Identify various physician orders that require clarification.

As a practical/vocational nurse, you will be an active member of the healthcare team. Utilizing the nursing process, you will be interacting with your patients, and they will rely on your competent skills and abilities. You will have many responsibilities, and you will be accountable for your actions.

The nurse is legally accountable for nursing practice according to the laws of the Nurse Practice Act. You will be responsible for providing quality nursing care based on a certain standard of care. This means that the care you give should be on the same level or quality that is reasonably expected from other nurses with comparable experience and training in a similar situation.

Legal awareness refers to the regulations and laws that govern the practice of nursing. Ethics are rules that deal with appropriate conduct and are concerned with moral responsibility and obligations. The National Association for Practical Nurse Education and Service (NAPNES) has developed standards of practice that serve as guidelines for responsible practical/vocational nursing. They appear in Appendix C.

Your knowledge of the legal and ethical aspects of your nursing practice will assist you in making appropriate decisions to protect you from lawsuits and legal charges.

NURSE PRACTICE ACTS/LICENSURE

The Nurse Practice Act is the most important law affecting your professional nursing practice. Each state has a Nurse Practice Act that authorizes the formulation of a state board of nursing. The board is created to develop and enforce rules and regulations concerning the practice of nursing, and it is bound by the laws of the act. The Nurse Practice Act is law and can only be changed by the state legislature.

It should be noted that some states have separate Nurse Practice Acts for practical/vocational nurses and for registered nurses. Usually the Act will define the practice of nursing, registered or practical/vocational, based on the specific scope of practice and the educational requirements. In addition to defining the practice of nursing, the Nurse Practice Act establishes the qualifications needed to practice nursing, specifies the rules and regulations for licensure, determines the state nursing board's authority, and specifies the makeup of the board and how that board will function. The Act may also include certain violations that may result in disciplinary actions by the board. In the majority of states, the board members are appointed by the governor. As discussed earlier, some states have separate acts for L.P.N.'s/L.V.N.'s and R.N.'s; and some states also have separate nursing boards.

Interpreting the Nurse Practice Act can be complex and difficult. The wording tends to be broad and can vary from state to state. Basically, the Act is established to assist the nurse in remaining within the legal scope of practice in the particular state. It is not a verbatim statement of all the things you are able to do in your nursing practice. Therefore, nurses must rely upon their knowledge, skills, educational preparation, and hospital procedures and policies in the performace of nursing duties.

Specific problems can arise in the interpretation of the Nurse Practice Act. For example, the Act dictates that the nurse has a legal duty to carry out the orders given by a dentist or physician. As a licensed nurse, there is also a legal and ethical duty and responsibility to use individual nursing judgment in the delivery of patient care. How do you obey orders and still act independently? When you believe the order is incorrect, the physician should be approached. If the physician does not clarify or correct the order, the immediate nursing supervisor should be notified. Difficulties of this nature can be handled administratively between nursing administration and the appropriate medical staff committees.

Occasionally, Nurse Practice Acts and hospital policy do not agree. Hospitals are required by hospital licensing laws to develop policies and procedures for their practice. The policies and procedures of the nursing department are established to determine permitted nursing practice within the facility. The scope of practice allowed within the facility cannot be broader than that outlined in the state Nurse Practice Act. It is important to remember that the facility cannot legally expand the scope of nursing practice. The nurse has a legal obligation to practice nursing within the confines of the law as stated in the Practice Act.

The *state board of nursing* is an agency created by provision of the Nurse Practice Act. The National Council of State Boards of Nursing, Inc., founded in 1978, is composed of at least sixty Member Boards of Nursing. This organization is responsible for preparing the licensing examinations for nurses: the National Council Licensure Examination for Registered Nurses (NCLEX-RN) and its counterpart for practical/vocational nurses, the National Council Licensure Examination for Practical Nurses (NCLEX-PN). Responsibilities of the board include:

- Rules and regulations for administering the Nurse Practice Act.
- Review applications for licensure.
- Issue licenses to qualified applicants.
- Develop standards for nursing programs.
- Nursing program approval.
- Renewal of nurses' licenses.
- Develop standards for licensure examinations.
- Monitor state board licensure examinations.
- Review charges of improper conduct by nurses.
- Make appropriate disciplinary actions as provided by the Act.

The members of the board are usually appointed by the governor; the board can range in size from seven to seventeen members. Members represent the nursing profession; in some states, a public member and a physician member are mandated.

Licensure

The basic qualifications for licensure may include graduation from an approved basic nursing education program, fluency in the English language, good moral character, good physical and mental health, high school diploma or equivalent, and attainment of minimum age. The state board of nursing has the responsibility for developing standards for the approval of nursing programs. Nursing schools must meet the requirements of the standards in order for their graduates to take the state board examination for licensure. The NCLEX-PN examination is discussed in Chapter Ten on career awareness.

A *license,* or permission to practice, is given when the applicant meets the requirements of state law and the state board of nursing. Unless the license is revoked or suspended, it remains valid. Continuing education requirements for maintaining licensure is discussed in Chapter Ten. *Registration* is the listing or registering of the license with the state for a fee. The license must be registered with the state in which the nurse practices before the nurse can legally practice. Renewal of the license is in accordance with the laws of each state.

Licensure by *endorsement* refers to acceptance of a previously issued state license by another state without additional requirements. Some states do require that a nurse moving into the state meet the requirements for new licensure. A state may require a nurse to meet other criteria before granting a license to practice by endorsement. For the correct information, write to the board of nursing of the state in which you are interested. State and Territorial Boards of Nursing and Practical Nursing are listed in Appendix A of this text.

LEGAL ASPECTS: TYPES OF LAWS

Statutory laws are enacted by the legislature at the county, city, state, or federal level. Nurse Practice Acts are statutory laws because each state has the power to pass laws that regulate the nursing profession. Laws enacted by legislative bodies carry the greatest weight in the court.

Common laws are derived from previous judicial decisions, common usage, or custom. After a judiciary decision is made, it establishes precedent for interpretation of the law in cases involving similar circumstances. Common law prevents the usage of different sets of rules to judge different people when circumstances are similar.

Criminal law defines a crime as a wrong committed against a person or property; the crime is also considered to be committed against the public or to affect the public welfare. Crimes are punishable by removal of privileges, parole, imprisonment, or fines.

Civil laws regulate the conduct of activities between individuals or businesses. A *tort* is a wrong committed by a person against another person or his property. Individuals and businesses may bring legal action against others when there is a breach of civil law. Judicial decisions in these cases are intended to correct the wrongful situation and may include payment of monies to parties involved.

LEGAL ISSUES

The law requires nurses to provide safe and competent care. This is defined as the level of care that would be rendered by a comparable nurse in a similar circumstance and is referred to as a standard of care. Nurses are prepared to deliver the appropriate standard of care through theory and clinical training. Basic legal issues of concern are discussed here.

Negligence occurs when a person fails to perform as a reasonably prudent person would have performed in a similar circumstance. Requirements to establish negligence include:

1. A standard of care.
2. A breach of duty or failure to meet the standard of care.
3. Damages or injury resulting from the breach of duty.
4. The injury or damage must be the result of the nurse's negligent act.

Malpractice is also negligence. It refers to negligence by the professional person with a license. Consequently, malpractice is used to describe negligence by nurses in the performance of their duties. Taking the wrong action and failing to act reasonably both constitute negligence.

Invasion of privacy takes two forms, the physical and the confidential. All information regarding a patient belongs to that patient. Only those people who are involved in the patient's care and who have a need to know should be allowed access to the patient's medical chart. The information provided by patients to the healthcare team is of a personal nature. Because it is privileged communication, it should not be shared with others without the patient's consent. A nurse who gives out information without authorization from the patient or the legal guardian can be held liable.

Patients have the right to physical privacy during the administration of nursing and medical care. Physical privacy can be provided by making sure that the patient is appropriately draped for procedures, closing the door of the room, drawing the curtain around the bed, and restricting visitors. A student who is interested in a particular procedure or treatment being administered to a patient should obtain the patient's permission through the clinical instructor.

Defamation of character is defined as any false written or oral statement that damages the reputation of another. Written defamation is called *libel,* and oral defamation is called *slander.*

Charting on the patient's medical record should be objective and factual. Nurses who chart their opinions, such as "patient is addictive" or "patient is rude," could be held liable for defamation of character.

Assault is a threat or an attempt to do something that makes a person believe that he or she will be touched without giving permission. *Battery* is the unlawful touching or unconsented touching of a person. Battery is the assault carried out through physical contact.

An example of assault is: "If you don't stay in bed, we will have to put you in restraints." The restraints may never be applied, but the patient has the fear that they may be, and so the nurse could be liable for assault.

Examples of battery include forcing a patient to take medications or to submit to a treatment or procedure. Patients have the right to refuse medical treatment and care, even if the care and treatment are beneficial to their well-being. Implied consent is appropriate. For example, if the nurse has an injection for the patient and he positions himself appropriately to receive the medication, battery cannot be charged against the nurse.

Preventing movement or making a person stay in a place without his consent is *false imprisonment.* The means can be physical or nonphysical. Nonphysical means would include removing the patient's clothes to prevent him from leaving the hospital. All persons have the right to make decisions for themselves. If the patient wants to do something that is against medical treatment, efforts should be made to help the person understand and comply with the treatment plan. However, if the patient still disagrees, then the appropriate documentation should be made in the patient's chart. This documentation should include the patient instruction and education regarding the issue, the persons notified, and the policies followed to protect the patient, the nurse, and the facility.

Patients cannot be restricted from leaving the hospital for nonpayment of a bill. Refusing discharge would constitute false imprisonment.

In the psychiatric setting, particular laws apply. Some patients are admitted voluntarily, and the restrictions on false imprisonment that apply to patients in the general acute care level also apply to these patients. Those patients who are admitted involuntarily require specific techniques for confinement. These measures are determined by law and by the policy of the individual institution. Nurses who work with psychiatric patients must know the laws and policies governing the use of restraints in patient care.

LEGAL DOCUMENTS

The Medical Chart

The patient's medical record or hospital chart is sometimes referred to as the *medical chart*. This document is a written history of the patient's illness, a record of observations made, decisions reached, and care given. It can be used as evidence of what occurred and what was done for the patient. Charting must be accurate and complete to provide evidence of the quality of care given to the patient. When patient observations or nursing care are not charted, the legal assumption is that they did not occur. Additionally, entries in the medical record must be written objectively and legibly. Appropriate notations can protect you from liability for the actions of others by showing that you followed appropriate procedures and timely notification of proper personnel.

Purposes of the Medical Chart

Data Collection for Research.   Information from patient medical records may contribute to the statistics of various research projects. Only authorized persons can have access to patient records. Permission must be obtained to use patient medical charts. When the medical chart is used for research, for various audits, or by students for class assignments, the identity of the patient must be concealed by using only the initials or assigned numbers. When this is not done, healthcare providers and those involved risk legal issues regarding the patient's right to privacy.

Provides Continuity of Care.   Patient care is administered by various members of the healthcare team. It is vital to have communication among the team members concerning the patient care treatment plan, patient response to the treatment given, decisions for further care, patient progress, and any necessary modification of the treatment regime. Sharing information among the healthcare workers caring for the patient can prevent duplication and assists in reducing errors.

Legal Document/Permanent Record of Patient's Care.   The medical record is a written account of the patient's hospitalization and the care administered. Entries are always dated and timed; nursing notes cover the total period of the hospital stay in a sequential manner on a twenty-four-a-day basis. The medical record is filed and maintained for future needs and is admissible in courts of law. The nurse's individual personal beliefs should not be included when recording and interpreting observations. Any person who signs an entry on the chart can be called as a witness should the patient's chart be involved in a legal action.

Wills

People often delay initiating or revising a will until they become ill. Some hospitals require that the nursing supervisor or the business office be contacted to handle the legal procedures. Frequently, the nurse may be asked to serve as a witness. There are some suggested guidelines when witnessing the signing of a will:

- The witness should see the person during the signing of the will, and the two should sign in the presence of one another.
- The witness should believe that the person signing the will is aware of what he is doing and is not under the influence of medications that would affect his mentality.
- The person acting as a witness should feel that the person signing the will is doing so voluntarily without pressure.
- The witness needs to make certain that the document is indeed a will.
- Persons receiving benefits from a will are not eligible to act as a witness to the signing of the will.

Consent Forms

Patients have the right to participate in decisions regarding their medical care. They have the right to refuse treatment, care, and procedures. To protect the patient's rights, consent forms are obtained before any treatment is administered. The only exception to this rule is a medical emergency in which the patient's life is in danger. The responsibility for obtaining consent for medical treatment is on the physician. A written, signed consent is generally preferred in order to have a record and proof of consent. Consent must be voluntary and informed. *Voluntary* means that the patient is providing consent of her own free will. *Informed* means that the patient is aware of the type of treatment planned, the risks involved, and the alternatives to treatment in order to make a reasonable decision.

Who May Sign Consents? The confusion over who may sign consents is longstanding. A competent adult consents to her own medical treatment and care. A competent person has the ability to understand the matter under consideration and the consequences of making decisions. An adult is a person eighteen years or older or a person who has entered a valid marriage, even if the marriage has been dissolved.

Spouses do not have the legal right to sign for the patient. If the patient is an incompetent adult, no nonemergency care or medical treatment may be given until consent is obtained from the legal guardian.

Persons under the age of eighteen are considered minors and do not have the legal right to consent to medical treatment and care. If the parents are divorced, usually consent is obtained from the parent who has custody of the child.

The emancipated minor of sixteen years of age or older, who lives away from the home of the parent or guardian, and who manages his or her own financial affairs can give consent for care and treatment without guardian or parent consent or knowledge. Other minors who have legal authority to consent to medical treatment are those on active duty with the military services and married minors. In some states, minors receiving treatment for pregnancy, those who are victims of sexual assault, those who have reportable communicable diseases, and those over age twelve with a drug or alcohol problem can provide consent for treatment and care.

It is important for the nurse to be familiar with the hospital's consent manual regarding individual hospital and state policies and laws in specific situations.

Admissions Agreement

This agreement describes the type of care the hospital provides for the patient and includes the patient's responsibility to assume costs for the care provided. The document discusses responsibility for the patient's personal belongings and valuables, outlines the patient's financial obligation, and provides for the release of information to various agencies for payment purposes.

Releases

A release is a type of legal document used to excuse a party from responsibility or liability. An example of a release that is commonly used in hospitals is the side rails release. Hospitals require that a patient sign this release if the patient refuses to use side rails. The form states that the patient is aware of the possible dangers of not using the side rails and that he will not hold the hospital responsible for any injury that may occur as a result of not using them.

Another common release used in hospitals, is the "Discharge Against Medical Advice." When a patient demands to leave the hospital without a discharge order from the authorizing physician, the patient is requested to sign a "Discharge Against Medical Advice" release. The physician or the nurse should talk to the patient and explain why continued hospitalization is needed. If the patient still wants to leave, then the release form is completed and the patient's signature is obtained. The form states that the hospital is released from responsibility for the patient's condition because he or she left the hospital against medical advice. If the patient refuses to sign, this should be noted and witnessed. When the patient leaves the hospital against medical advice, most hospitals require that the physician in charge, the nursing supervisor, and hospital administration be notified.

Incident Reports

Patient incident reports are completed when there is a patient accident or an error in treatment or medication. The form is completed for the intended use of the hospital attorney. The hospital personnel who are most familiar with the incident should complete the incident report following hospital guidelines and policies. The report will require full details related to the incident—date, time, place of occurrence, age and sex of the patient, physician's name, and the date of form completion. Some forms provide for the details of the incident as related by the patient and may include a space for any witnesses to the incident. The incident report is not a part of the patient's chart. It is usually routed to the nursing administration office or to another designated administrative department.

WITNESS/EXPERT WITNESS

As a healthcare team member, nurses may be asked to testify in court about a specific case. It is not necessary to be a part of a lawsuit to be asked to testify in court. As an expert witness, the nurse is asked to testify because of education, expertise, or experience in a particular area of nursing. It is not necessary that the expert witness know any of the particulars of the individual case. The purpose of the the expert witness's testimony is to make certain complex and highly technical material clearer for the jury. The ordinary witness provides testimony about information that has been observed or heard.

The nurse may be a voluntary or involuntary witness. As an involuntary witness, the nurse may be required to testify when one of the parties in the case requests the court to issue a subpoena. A subpoena is a legal document that requires a person to appear in court at a certain date and time for the purpose of providing testimony in a certain case.

REDUCING THE RISK OF MALPRACTICE CLAIMS _____

As a healthcare professional, the nurse has a legal responsibility for individual practice. Ethically, the nurse is involved in efforts to develop and maintain conditions of employment that are conducive to high-quality nursing care. Listed below are some of the reasons for patient litigations.

Reasons for Patient Litigation

- Improper use of equipment or supplies.
- Inappropriate performance of a procedure.
- Failure by the nurse to follow a physician's order correctly and in a timely manner.
- Lack of protection from falls and other injuries.
- Failure by the nurse to make timely, accurate entries in the medical record.
- Lack of appropriate patient observation and monitoring.
- Failure to function within the area of expertise and job description.
- Inappropriate administration of medications.
- Unexpected change in the patient's condition or an unexpected outcome.
- Loss of rapport or poor rapport with hospital personnel.

Guidelines to Reduce Risks

Know Your Job Description.   Hospitals and healthcare agencies have various job descriptions for different position levels. It is important to know the limitations and expectations of your job as defined by the agency's policies.

Remain Alert.   Make every attempt to remain focused when working and communicating with patients and families. Each part of your job demands your full energy and attention.

Read Your Policy and Procedure Manual.   As nursing changes, it will be necessary to maintain currency in policies and procedures. The manual should be realistic and should cover actual nursing practice within the hospital or agency.

Chart Objectively, Timely, Accurately, and Completely.
Make chart entries promptly and label late entries. Make certain that you follow the agency's policy. Be specific and avoid conclusions; chart observations, signs, and symptoms. Make charting corrections carefully and use appropriate procedure.

Review Your Performance Appraisal.
Be aware of your weaknesses and strengths in nursing practice. Determine the appropriate means of resolution for weaknesses that have been identified.

Report Incidents.
Make sure that incident reports are completed in a timely fashion and routed to the designated office. All lines should be completely filled in as directed. If certain questions are not applicable, follow the agency's policy for notation. In some institutions, simply write NA to show that a question that was not answered was not overlooked.

Establish and Maintain Rapport With Patients.
Patients need to feel in control of themselves and prefer to be included in decisions about their care and treatment. Communicating with patients about their treatment plan and showing your concern for the outcome of the care is important in maintaining patient rapport.

Be Involved in Nursing Practice Evaluation.
The nursing audit process is an objective tool for evaluating nursing care and provides a mechanism for identifying needed change. Regular audits will show if personnel are in compliance with current hospital policy and procedures. Be actively involved in determining the appropriate action required to bring nursing care up to the standards of expectation.

Question Certain Orders For Patient and Legal Protection.
Nurse–patient relationships are important. Communication between the patient and the nurse facilitates an effective working relationship necessary for the intended outcome of the patient's treatment plan. Even though the nurse may be certain of the orders, especially medication orders, if the patient questions an order, it is prudent to wait and check for clarification.

Question and Clarify Orders When The Patient's Condition Changes.
Nurses are to report any significant changes in the patient's condition to the physician. It is reasonable and prudent to do this even if the physician does not request the information. It is possible that some medication or treatment may be affecting the patient's condition adversely and should be discontinued, at least, until the orders can be clarified.

When you are inexperienced with standing physician orders, contact the supervisor and the physician for clarification and guidance. The law prevents nurses from "practicing medicine" without a license, but it does require that nurses exercise judgment about patient conditions. When nurses follow standing orders, they are not practicing medicine, but they are exercising nursing judgment.

Take Special Precautions With Verbal Orders. To reduce the risk of miscommunication when taking telephone and verbal orders, document all actions taken and the conversation with the physician. The following guidelines may prove helpful:

- Write down what you will be telling the physician and keep your note available for reference. Include the details of the situation.
- Note the time, date, and the physician's name.
- Read the orders back to the physician, slowly. Make certain to document that the orders were read back to the physician, and that the physician verified them as read.

All ambiguous orders should be questioned. Follow the agency's policy and procedure for clarifying ambiguous or inappropriate orders. Make certain that your actions are documented.

Nurses are expected to question orders that do not follow "common" or "normal" practice. When the nurse reports patient symptoms accurately, documents correctly, makes sure that appropriate orders are followed, and questions unclear or inappropriate orders, then legal risks are reduced.

MALPRACTICE INSURANCE

Healthcare professionals disagree as to whether a nurse should carry individual malpractice insurance. Some experts believe that having malpractice insurance simply invites lawsuits. These experts also believe that the best protection against litigation is quality nursing practice.

It can also be argued that malpractice insurance is a "must" for all nurses, regardless of the area of clinical practice. Additionally, some nurses find it comforting to have their own attorney. The belief here is that the agency's attorney will be representing the agency and protecting the agency's interest, not the nurse's. Whatever your preference, make sure you investigate carefully.

Some hospitals and healthcare agencies carry liability insurance for the employer and the employee. Based on the limitations of the policy, liability insurance will cover the costs of legal counsel and provide protection in the case of judgment or settlement.

Nurses may obtain liability insurance from several companies through various professional organizations or by dealing with the insurance company directly. Many companies advertise through various professional magazines, and the application for membership is often included as a part of the advertisement. Mass marketing has been very effective in helping to keep the premiums for nurses' liability insurance at a reasonable cost.

How much coverage should you buy? A difficult question at best. Some insurance carriers no longer offer a $500,000 policy because of the larger settlements now being awarded and report that nurses are requesting a $1,000,000 to $1,500,000 policies. The costs range from approximately $50 to $100 per year. It certainly pays to shop wisely. It is imporant to remember that these costs will rise with inflation. Some nursing specialists such as nurse midwives, nurse anesthetists, and nurse practitioners are required to pay increased costs for their liability insurance.

Malpractice policies for nurses are somewhat similar in the basics, but there are some differences. For example, a liability policy may include personal liability coverage. This means that the nurse will be covered for nonnursing incidents. Take a good look at individual policies; when analyzing policies, ask yourself these questions:

- What are the financial limitations of the policy?
- Who is covered?
- Under what conditions is the policy renewable?
- What is the annual premium cost?
- How long does the coverage last? *Occurrence coverage* refers to coverage for any incidents that occurred while the policy was in effect, even if a suit is filed after the policy has lapsed. *Claims-made coverage* means that coverage is provided only if the claim is filed while the policy is in effect.
- When am I covered? On the job and off the job?
- Am I provided with an attorney? This does not mean that you get to choose the attorney or to decide when you need one. The insurance company will make those decisions.
- Is my salary guaranteed when I am in court?
- Are all the defense costs covered?
- Am I required to settle?
- What other items are included in the coverage?

When you purchase your insurance coverage, be sure to read the policy and make sure you understand all issues. There are some important things to remember. If you change your position or status, the insurer should be notified in writing, and you should keep a copy of the notification letter on file. Be sure to inform your company of any incidents you are involved in that may lead to litigation. You may also call and request advice about an incident or an issue that requires clarification. When you telephone, be sure to have your policy number available and make a note of whom you spoke with, what was said, and the date and the time of the conversation. Any written correspondence should always include your name and policy number.

Should you decide to cancel your policy, simply return the policy and notify the company by letter, with the date that you want the coverage to end.

Before you purchase malpractice insurance, ask several companies for brochures and a copy of their policy for your review. This will let you do some comparison shopping. It is well worth the time to find the company that provides you with the coverage that makes you feel protected and comfortable.

REVIEW/DISCUSSION/ACTIVITIES

1. List at least seven responsibilities of the state board of practical/vocational nursing.
2. What are the requirements to establish negligence?
3. What are the purposes of the medical chart?
4. Some reasons for patient litigation are given in this chapter. Provide examples of each reason listed.
5. List and discuss the guidelines to reduce risk of lawsuits.

BIBLIOGRAPHY

Brent, E. A. "Think! . . . Before You Witness That Will." *RN Magazine* 43 (1980): 61, 64.

Grippando, G. M. *Nursing Perspectives and Issues,* 3d ed. Albany, N.Y.: Delmar, 1986.

Hemelt, M. D., and Mackert, M.E. *Dynamics of Law in Nursing and Health Care,* 2d ed. Reston, Va.: Reston Publishing, 1987.

Mandell, M. "Ten Legal Commandments for Nurses Who Get Sued." *Nursing Life* 6 (1986): 19–21.

CHAPTER

8

Nursing Ethics

Ethics consists of rules or guidelines concerned with appropriate conduct and actions. They represent judgments about moral responsibility and obligations. Some professions, including, medicine, law, and nursing, have written statements of their beliefs about what constitutes ethical behavior by their members. Members of professions have a particularly specialized knowledge and expertise that is used to make critical decisions affecting the lives of other people, and the purpose of code of ethics is to describe the correct and moral way to use this power.

The National Association for Practical Nurse Education and Service (NAPNES) has developed standards of practice that serve as guidelines for responsible practical/vocational nursing practice. They appear in Appendix C.

Nursing is a vital service provided to your patients. It is based on trust that the nurse will do what is correct and required to benefit the patient. Concerns about what is right or wrong have always been with us, and various ethical issues relating to current times demand scrupulous examination.

Today, societal factors and our social values are changing rapidly. Additionally, there is a consistent advancement of technology that quickly brings problems and issues before us. Many of the concerns are emotionally charged and require intensive debate and discussion.

There can be conflict in values, problem resolution, professional judgment, and professional options. Today's practical/vocational nurse is confronted by ethical decisions that can have significant and long-term implications. Nurses have specialized knowledge and skills that they use to make decisions affecting their patients. In these very complex matters they must know what their legal rights are, as well as the rights of the patient. Figure 8-1 shows "A Patient's Bill of Rights" as adopted by the American Hospital Association.

In seeking a better understanding for themselves, nurses consider all aspects of an issue. The professional values are shaped by the strength of the personal values.

Figure 8–1 A Patient's Bill of Rights. *Courtesy the American Hospital Association, 840 North Lake Shore Drive, Chicago, IL 60611. Copyright 1975. All rights reserved.*

This policy document presents the official position of the American Hospital Association as approved by the Board of Trusstees and House of Delegates.

The American Hospital Association presents a Patient's Bill of Rights with the expectation that observance of these rights will contribute to

continued

more effective patient care and greater satisfaction for the patient, his physician, and the hospital organization. Further, the Association presents these rights in the expectation that they will be supported by the hospital on behalf of its patients, as an integral part of the healing process. It is recognized that a personal relationship between the physician and the patient is essential for the provision of proper medical care. The traditional physician-patient relationship takes on a new dimension when care is rendered within an organizational structure. Legal precedent has established that the institution itself also has a responsibility to the patient. It is in recognition of these factors that these rights are affirmed.

1. The patient has the right to considerate and respectful care.
2. The patient has the right to obtain from his physician complete current information concerning his diagnosis, treatment, and prognosis in terms the patient can be reasonably expected to understand. When it is not medically advisable to give such information to the patient, the information should be made available to an appropriate person in his behalf. He has the right to know, by name, the physician responsible for coordinating his care.
3. The patient has the right to receive from his physician information necessary to give informed consent prior to the start of any procedure and/or treatment. Except in emergencies, such information for informed consent should include but not necessarily be limited to the specific procedure and/or treatment, the medically significant risks involved, and the probable duration of incapacitation. Where medically significant alternatives for care or treatment exist, or when the patient requests information concerning medical alternatives, the patient has the right to such information. The patient also has the right to know the name of the person responsible for the procedures and/or treatment.
4. The patient has the right to refuse treatment to the extent permitted by law and to be informed of the medical consequences of his action.
5. The patient has the right to every consideration of his privacy concerning his own medical care program. Case discussion, consultation, examination, and treatment are confidential and should be conducted discreetly. Those not directly involved in his care must have the permission of the patient to be present.
6. The patient has the right to expect that all communications and records pertaining to his care should be treated as confidential.
7. The patient has the right to expect that within its capacity a hospital must make reasonable response to the request of a patient for services. The hospital must provide evaluation, service, and/or referral as indicated by the urgency of the case. When medically

continued

permissible, a patient may be transferred to another facility only after he has received complete information and explanation concerning the needs for an alternatives to such a transfer. The institution to which the patient is to be transferred must first have accepted the patient for transfer.

8. The patient has the right to obtain information as to any relationship of his hospital to other health care and educational institutions insofar as his care is concerned. The patient has the right to obtain information as to the existence of any professional relationships among individuals, by name, who are treating him.

9. The patient has the right to be advised if the hospital proposes to engage in or perform human experimentation affecting his care or treatment. The patient has the right to refuse to participate in such research projects.

10. The patient has the right to expect reasonable continuity of care. He has the right to know in advance what appointment times and physicians are available and where. The patient has the right to expect that the hospital will provide a mechanism whereby he is informed by his physician or a delegate of the physician of the patient's continuing health care requirements following discharge.

11. The patient has the right to examine and receive an explanation of his bill regardless of source of payment.

12. The patient has the right to know what hospital rules and regulations apply to his conduct as a patient.

No catalog of rights can guarantee for the patient the kind of treatment he has a right to expect. A hospital has many functions to perform, including the prevention and treatment of disease, the education of both health professionals and patients, and the conduct of clinical research. All these activities must be conducted with an overriding concern for the patient, and, above all, the recognition of his dignity as a human being. Success in achieving this recognition assures success in the defense of the rights of the patient.

During the 1970s the American Hospital Association's Board of Trustees had a Committee on Health Care for the Disadvantaged, which developed the *Statement on a Patient's Bill of Rights*. That document was approved by the AHA House of Delegates on February 6, 1973, and has been published in various forms. This reprinting and reclassification conforms with the current classification system for AHA documents. The contents are unchanged.

MAKING ETHICAL DECISIONS

Making difficult, complex ethical decisions is an inherent part of the practical/vocational nurse's role. The decisions can involve identifying the rights of the individual patient, respecting those rights, and performing specific duties that protect the patient's rights. Figure 8-2 is the Code

Figure 8–2   Code of Ethics for Practical/Vocational Nurses. *Courtesy the National Association for Practical Nurse Education and Service, Inc.*

The Licensed Practical/Vocational Nurse Shall:

1. Consider as a basic obligation the conservation of life and the prevention of disease.

2. Promote and protect the physical, mental, emotional and spiritual health of the patient and his family.

3. Fulfill all duties faithfully and efficiently.

4. Function within established legal guidelines.

5. Accept personal responsibility (for his/her acts) and seek to merit the respect and confidence of all members of the health team.

6. Hold in confidence all matters coming to his/her knowledge, in the practice of his/her profession, and in no way and at no time violate this confidence.

7. Give conscientious service and charge just remuneration.

8. Learn and respect the religious and cultural beliefs of his/her patient and of all people.

9. Meet his/her obligation to the patient by keeping abreast of current trends in health care through reading and continuing education.

10. As a citizen of the United States of America, uphold the laws of the land and seek to promote legislation that will meet the health needs of its people.

Copyright © 1987 by NAPNES (1400 Spring Street, Suite 310, Silver Spring, Maryland 20910, (301) 588-2491)

of Ethics for the licensed practical/vocational nurse developed by The National Association for Practical Nurse Education and Service.

Ethical conduct is an individual and personal matter since we each have our own view of what is right and what is wrong. Nurses must be aware of their own values and must be nonjudgmental in making decisions about their patients. The following approach might be used when making ethical decisions:

Clarify and Reaffirm Your Own Values

Frequently, we do not assess our values until we are faced with a difficult decision. Clarifying our values is a continuous growth process, and it is to be expected that our position on certain issues may change as this growth process takes place. Having a clear undertanding of our own values helps us choose among various alternatives and options. It also helps us explain and validate our decisions and actions to others. It is important to remember that the patient may make a choice that differs from your opinion or belief. As a patient advocate, the nurse must support the patient's right to make individual choices.

Obtain All the Facts

Try to determine what the patient knows about his condition and how he feels about the situation. Learn everything you can about the patient's medical condition, various treatment alternatives, and the prognosis.

Look for Guidelines

Make every attempt to clarify legal and professional obligations. Discuss the issue with the nursing administration department or your agency's legal department. These departments are excellent resources and can provide assistance in gathering the facts. You may choose to consult your own legal counsel. Read your agency's policy manual for clarification of their position on the particular issue. Some hospitals have ethics commit-tees that can provide support and guidance. Hospital pastoral department representatives can not only offer emotional support but can also provide assistance in clarifying some moral issues associated with ethical dilem-mas.

Determine the Various Alternatives

Review each alternative, along with its consequences. Ethical dilemmas are often complicated because no one solution may be correct. Try to determine the actions that offer the best solution for all involved.

Choose a Position

It is necessary to support your position with clear thinking and reasoning. You nurse must be comfortable with an individual decision, which is a supportive basis for explaining your actions should this be required or requested.

FACTORS AFFECTING ETHICAL DECISION MAKING _____

Religious Beliefs

For many people, religious beliefs form the basis for making ethical decisions. On certain occasions, nurses may choose to make decisions based on the particular issue at hand, regardless of the religious doctrine of their religion or church.

Nurses are encouraged to seek employment in those hospitals and agencies whose policies and practices complement their basic beliefs. This reduces the potential for conflict between nurses and agency administration.

Patient Rights

The patient should be allowed to express his feelings about his condition. As a patient advocate, the nurse should assist the patient in obtaining answers to his questions about his condition, prognosis, and treatment. The American Nurses' Association Code of Ethics states that each patient has the right to:

- decide what treatment he will refuse or accept.
- receive the information he needs to make an informed decision.
- be warned of the possible side effects of different treatments.

Cultural Beliefs

Each culture has a value system and attitudes about human life. It is imperative that the nurse respect human individuality. This is a difficult and complex issue at times because the patient's cultural beliefs may not be in keeping with current nursing practice.

Technological Advances

Many significant ethical issues have arisen as a result of the advancement of medical technology. The prolongation of life through mechanical means has confronted the healthcare profession with the ''quality of life'' issue. Additionally, the sophisticated technology brings to the forefront the need for a universal definition of life and death.

Finances

Numerous questions are being asked about the spending of monies for healthcare provision. What should a healthcare system provide? What fees should be charged? Should everyone pay for the services? Who is eligible for care? The technological advances discussed above can be included here. Many of the mechanical devices are very costly, and not everyone can afford the services. Sometimes, there is a limited amount of equipment available, and the difficult decision must be made as to who is eligible to receive treatment. These difficult and complex decisions can have far-reaching effects.

Legal Implications

It is clear that nurses must perform their responsibilities according to their respective Nurse Practice Acts. Many ethical issues confronted by practical/vocational nurses have legal implications.

Strong societal attitudes have been the impetus to incorporate certain ideas into law. An example is the action taken as a response to the needs of the handicapped. Businesses and public facilities have allocated vehicle parking places, curbsides have been built to accommodate wheelchairs, and numerous policies have been written to bring about needed change.

Another example of change due to society's attitudes is the abortion issue. Many years ago, abortions were against the law. Many physicians saw the end result of abortions done under poor conditions and were so moved that they chose to perform them. The laws were thus changed as a result of public attitudes.

Employ Status

A nurse's economic well being is important. When making ethical decisions, there are certain considerations and loyalties to the employer. Codes of ethics for nurses dictate that patient concern be foremost. In day-to-day nursing practice, there is also concern for personal economic and career loss should the nurse's decision affect the employer in a negative way. These serious concerns can add stress to an already difficult situation.

SPECIFIC ETHICAL ISSUES IN NURSING

Mechanical Life Support

Medical technological advancement frequently gives us the ability to delay death. The controversial question is, should death be delayed? Another important question is, what is death? The answers vary from state to state.

Patients frequently sign a living will, asking that no extraordinary means be utilized to sustain life. When this in effect, a no-code order must be written by the physician on the patient's medical chart. Questions surrounding life support include: When should life support measures be initiated? When should they be terminated? What is "extraordinary"? The issue is emotionally charged, and the decisions can be very difficult. When caring for a terminally ill patient on life support, the nurse must be aware of state laws regarding the definition of death and the legally binding nature of living wills.

Definition of Death. Generally, the cessation of brain wave activity recorded on an electroencephalogram (EEG) for a period of time establishes the patient as brain dead. However, mechanical life support systems can be used to maintain circulatory and respiratory functions.

Organ Transplants

The Uniform Anatomical Gift Act allows anyone over age eighteen to sign a donor card, willing some or all of his organs after death. The number of transplants is increasing because of improvements in tissue typing, improved surgical techniques, and increased success with immunologic suppressant medications.

When organ transplant is a viable option for the patient, one must carefully consider the taking of organs from one person's body to save or improve the quality of another's life. The well-being and quality of life of both the donor and the recipient must be considered. The decision can depend on a person's social, cultural, and religious beliefs and values.

While there is an increasing public awareness of successful organ transplants, body mutilation before or after death is an expressed concern. Other ethical questions raised include: How should the resources be assigned? For example, who gets the kidney or heart, the infant or the ailing research scientist? Who decides? How should the financial resources be allocated? Should thousands of dollars continue to be spent in experimental transplants, or would the funds be better spent on the current identified needs of the population? Who decides?

The nurse's role in this issue includes answering questions and referring patients and families to someone who can answer if the nurse is unable to. Obtaining consent for organ transplant is a medical responsibility, but the nurse can assist as with any other surgical procedure. Provide objective information and all available resources so that patients and families can make informed decisions about providing and receiving transplants.

Issues Related to Birth

Sexually active children, abortion, sterilization, artificial insemination, and test tube conception involve controversy and complex ethical issues. These issues have moral and legal implications. Religious doctrines and teaching have direct influence on healthcare workers and their patients. A brief examination of each of these issues can raise several questions for consideration.

Sexually Active Children. Persons under the age of eighteen may be sexually active and may need health care for a variety of reasons.

In some states, parents are required to provide consent for treatment, while in others, parental consent and knowledge are not necessary. Some healthcare workers, because of their own moral values, may find this situation difficult.

Abortion.   There are laws regulating abortions, but the controversy continues. Pro-life groups believe in fetal rights. They believe that these rights begin at the time of conception, and they favor restricting or eliminating maternal choice. The pro-choice groups believe that maternal rights should come first, and they favor abortion as an alternative to unwanted pregnancy.

Sterilization.   There are many reasons people consider sterilization. Couples may fear giving birth to a defective baby, they may decide to limit the number of children in the family, or they may choose not to have any children. Sometimes the male will undergo a vasectomy or the female will have a tubal ligation. For the most part, these procedures are irreversible. Religious and moral beliefs play an important role in making these decisions.

Artificial Insemination, Test Tube Conception.   Alternate means of conception may be a viable option for couples for a variety of reasons.

In test tube conception, the egg from the female is placed in a test tube with the sperm from her husband. The fertilized egg is then implanted in the female's uterus. Some believe that this is an unnatural way for conception to take place. Another issue of concern here is that the unused fertilized eggs are discarded.

In artificial insemination, the sperm donor may be the woman's husband or another man. The sperm or the fertilized egg is implanted in the female's uterus, who may be the donor's wife or another woman. When the woman is someone other than the donor's wife, she is referred to as a surrogate mother. Ethical, religious, and legal questions are raised in this issue. What are the legal rights of the surrogate mother? What are the rights of the man and woman? Is there an issue of adultery? Who gets legal custody and visiting rights if the couple divorce?

No-Code and Slow-Code Orders

When a person is terminally ill or death is imminent, the family, the physician, and sometimes the patient may decide that a no-code order is appropriate. The order is written and signed by the physician on the patient's medical chart. It is considered a legal order and is carried out when the patient goes into cardiac or respiratory arrest. It should be emphasized that the order must be written and signed by the physician. If a patient you did not attempt to resuscitate dies, and there is no written, signed no-code order, then healthcare workers, including the nurse, become legally liable.

Slow-code orders are not considered legal. Any unwritten, undocumented or documented, unsigned or unstated but "understood" no-code order is an illegal slow-code order. If the nurse carries out this order, and the patient dies due to lack of attempt to resuscitate, the nurse can be held legally liable. The only way to avoid the legal consequences of a slow-code order is to make sure that all no-code patients have a written, signed physician's order on the patient's medical chart.

Reporting an Incompetent Colleague

Reporting a colleague is never easy, but it is a responsibility to patients and a commitment to nursing ethics and conduct. When considering the issue, evaluate the situation carefully. Questions to consider may include: Has the conduct harmed a patient? Is it the result or the outcome that is being evaluated? Is the problem the incompetence or an ethical issue, or is it conduct with which you disagree? It is difficult at best to answer these questions, and the consequences of actions must be considered carefully.

These guidelines may prove helpful:

■ Always follow proper channels.
■ Be very specific and clear. Document the conduct and the issues.
■ Accuracy is a must. Describe only those things you know to be true.
■ Be open and consistent. Protect your credibility by including only those facts pertinent to the issue. State your account correctly and stand by it.
■ Document all actions taken. Be sure to include names, dates, times, places, purposes of meetings and discussions, and actions taken.
■ Continue to follow proper channels and procedures.

Before taking any actions against a colleague, it is advisable to discuss the situation with the colleague directly. Share your concern about the possible consequences of his or her conduct. If the outcome of your discussion is not satisfactory, then you may consult a trusted professional and follow an appropriate course of action.

The Chemically Abusive Nurse

A Nursing Task Force on Addiction and Psychological Disturbance was appointed by the American Nurses' Association in the early 1980s. The purpose of the task force was to develop guidelines for treatment and assistance for nurses whose alcoholism, drug abuse, or psychological problems interfere with their nursing practice. The guidelines were developed for use by state nurses' associations.

What are some of the behaviors or symptoms exhibited by the chemically abusive nurse? They may include:

- an increase in charting errors
- personality changes, mood swings
- changes in behavior and mental status
- inappropriate charting
- increased absenteeism and inability to meet scheduled work shifts
- unkempt appearance
- increased incidence of wasted or dropped medications when on duty
- complaints of poor pain control from assigned patients
- unsteady gait
- flushed face
- alcohol on the breath, slurred speech

Nursing has not always dealt with the problem of the chemically abusive nurse in an appropriate fashion. All too often, the nurse was transferred to another department, ignored, requested to leave the agency or hospital, or protected. Fortunately, nursing has become increasingly sensitive to the problem, and through professional associations, efforts are now devoted to providing the assistance necessary.

There are many factors that lead to chemical abuse by nurses. Included are frequent shift changes, staffing shortages, stress of nursing practice, unrealistic expectations of the profession, unrealistic personal expectations, frustration and anxiety, and inappropriate or missing self-care skills.

What should you do if you suspect that a nurse has this problem? First of all, do not confront the nurse. Make certain that a problem does exist. Gather information, including names, dates, times, and other pertinent data. Follow your agency's procedure and policies in this matter. In some institutions, the supervisor in charge is next in line to be notified. Other agencies have an ethics committee that can be contacted without fear of reprisal for the nurse reporting the incident. Once this step has been initiated, the committee or nursing administration will assume responsibility for the problem.

Investigation of the problem will continue, and if a problem does exist, appropriate actions will be taken. In some states, the needed referrals will be provided for the nurse involved. When you suspect a problem, ignoring or protecting a colleague is the worst ''favor'' you can give. Consider potential ramifications:

- job loss
- malpractice lawsuits
- harm to patients

- delays in getting treatment for the nurse involved
- disciplinary action by the licensing agency

Reporting a colleague is one of the most difficult and complex situations the nurse can encounter. It has personal and professional ramifications. However, it should be remembered that nursing must maintain its integrity and public trust. There are several qualities of a profession. One of the most significant is its ability to safeguard its standards of quality through self-monitoring.

Giving Medical Advice

Relatives and acquaintances may ask your opinion about certain treatments, medications, and healthcare providers. They believe in your expertise as a nurse, and they trust you to provide the most current information. Practical/vocational nurses must be careful about giving advice because of the responsibility assumed when answering off-the-job medical questions. The courts can hold a nurse responsible for healthcare advice given away from the work setting, especially when the person who is requesting the information makes it clear that he is asking for your professional opinion and has intentions of following your recommendations. The following guidelines are suggested for your legal protection when you encounter this situation:

- If you encounter an emergency, do what you can to help. Advise the person to seek emergency medical care immediately.
- Do not try to diagnose problems. It is safer to convince the person of all the reasons that they should not delay in seeking medical help.
- Avoid recommending a specific healthcare provider. Provide several names of providers or institutions and let the person make the decision.
- Do not criticize providers and institutions in the presence of others.
- If you are asked about a certain healthcare provider and you have reason to suspect the quality of care rendered, suggest getting a second opinion and provide the names of several other providers as suggested above.
- When you don't know something, admit it.
- Keep a record of what you say. Include names, dates, times, the event, other persons present, place, and exactly what was said.
- Stay current on first aid. Should an emergency arise, you would then be able to provide emergency care until medical help is available.
- Offer other resources for fielding questions, providing assistance, and suggesting referrals.

Those persons who seek your opinion in the off-duty setting value your expertise just as your patients do. Always remember, whether you are at work or not, you are still a nurse.

REVIEW/DISCUSSION/ACTIVITIES _____

1. What are the steps in making ethical decisions?
2. Bring in newspaper and magazine articles relating to ethical issues in healthcare or nursing. Discuss in class.
3. List the seven factors affecting ethical decision making.
4. Invite a nurse who has practiced for ten to fifteen years to come and discuss ethical issues relating to nursing practice ten to fifteen years ago. Compare the issues then and now.

BIBLIOGRAPHY _____

Creighton, Helen. *Law Every Nurse Should Know*, 4th ed. Philadelphia: W.B. Saunders Co., 1981.

Ellis, Janice, and Hartley, Celia. *Nursing in Today's World: Challenges, Issues, and Trends*, 3d ed. Philadelphia: J.B. Lippincott, 1988.

Fowler, M.D. "The Role of the Clinical Ethicist." *Heart Lung* 15 (May, 1986): 318–19.

Grippando, Gloria M. *Nursing Perspectives and Issues*, 3d ed. Albany, N.Y.: Delmar, 1986.

CHAPTER
9

Leadership/Association Membership

OBJECTIVES

The student successfully attaining the goals of this chapter will be able to:

- Identify qualities necessary for effective leadership/management.
- Describe management responsibilities in managing patient care and the patient unit.
- Name and discuss the nursing associations to which L.P./L.V.N.'s usually belong.
- Identify the guidelines for a successful mentoring relationship.
- Describe the advantages of networking.
- Describe two ways to communicate with your legislator.

The role of the licensed practical/vocational nurse has expanded in recent years. There are more areas of practice available to the practical/vocational nurse. Diagnosis-related group (DRGs) are impacting the patient's length of stay in the acute hospital. Consequently, many patients are discharged from the acute hospitals to the intermediate, skilled nursing, and long-term-care facilities, requiring a more sophisticated level of care. This has had an impact on the demand for licensed practical/vocational nurses with leadership and management skills in the intermediate and long term care facilities. Many nurses are recruited and hired for charge nurse and team leader positions.

Licensed practical/vocational nurses who are interested in these positions are expected to have additional educational preparation. Many employers require one to two years of staff level experience and personal qualities and skills supporting successful performance in a charge nurse or team leader position.

LEADERSHIP QUALITIES AND SKILLS

In clinical nursing practice, leadership positions for licensed practical/vocational nurses include charge nurse, team leader, and patient care coordinator. Whatever the position, certain qualities and skills are universally necessary for successful and effective leadership. The blueprint for success involves knowledge, leadership, and vision.

Knowledge includes the ability to manage in a growing, constantly challenging profession. Leadership refers to the ability to train others, and vision refers to the ability to follow established goals.

Qualities of an effective leader include being a good listener, fair, consistent, responsible, clinically and technically proficient, sensitive, open minded, emotionally mature, objective, and flexible.

Effective leaders promote teamwork and work cooperatively with others. They are emotionally mature and consistently maintain a professional atmosphere.

Practical/vocational nurses in leadership roles help others develop their skills by being willing to teach and share knowledge. This sharing of knowledge includes giving technical help and providing help with work problems.

The effective nurse leader welcomes open discussion and encourages others to express themselves. Nursing team members are encouraged to offer suggestions and make recommendations and are involved in the decision-making process.

The nurse leader is responsible, has good problem-solving abilities, and exhibits a consistent style of leadership. Additionally, the effective leader sets an appropriate example, remains flexible, and demonstrates a willingness to change.

The personal qualities of an effective leader can be developed and enhanced through academic preparation by attending leadership and management seminars and courses. Many providers of continuing education classes for nurses offer these courses.

MANAGEMENT RESPONSIBILITIES

Practical/vocational nurses in leadership roles are required to coordinate activities associated with patient care and nursing services. The effective nurse leader must also have management skills in directing patient care and managing the hospital unit.

The charge nurse or the team leader must be able to determine the nursing care required by the patients and to assess staff skills in order to make the appropriate assignments. Patient care must be planned so that patients will receive the care they require by the personnel with the skills to best provide that care. The patient care assignments are communicated to the nursing team members through the assignment sheet, which will include break and meal times along with other unit duties.

Evaluating the performance of the nursing team members assigned to the unit is also a responsibility of the charge nurse or the team leader. Provide written evaluations on a regular basis. Oral feedback is not enough. Schedule written evaluations regularly or according to the policy of the hospital in order to make them an expected and accepted part of the routine. Base your comments on the employee's performance on duties established by the job description.

Managing the hospital nursing unit includes providing necessary supplies and equipment, maintaining an environment that is safe for patients and unit personnel, and managing communication.

Frequently, charge nurses and team leaders will assign responsibility for supplies to a nursing team member or to the unit clerk. Medicines and equipment are ordered by the nurse assigned because of the responsibility involved.

The safety of the unit is the responsibility of the charge nurse or team leader. All nursing team members should be instructed in hospital safety and should report unsafe situations immediately. Many hospitals have preventive maintenance safety programs, and certain pieces of hospital equipment are checked at periodic intervals to maintain them in good working order. Unsafe conditions, such as spills or equipment in need of repair, should be reported to prevent falls and injuries.

Communication is an essential part of delivering patient care and managing the hospital unit. The practical/vocational nurse leader will be communicating with patients' family members and visitors. It is important to keep patient matters confidential. Some patient information is best provided by the patient's physician.

The team leader or charge nurse is responsible for keeping the physician informed about the patient's condition and response to care. Information must be accurate, clear, and complete. Information reported to the physician will often influence the physician's treatment plan for the patient.

The nursing supervisor is also responsible for the quality of care the patient receives. The charge nurse or team leader should keep the supervisor informed of unit activities and patient incidents. Written reports of all incidents should be forwarded to the nursing supervisor in a timely manner. To maintain an effective and positive working relationship with the supervisor, good communication is essential.

Effective nursing leadership is a key to the successful, well organized nursing team. The team leader or charge nurse, through effective working relationships with other healthcare team members, is in a strategic position to affect the quality of patient care.

NURSING ORGANIZATIONS

Involvement in professional organizations provides an opportunity for a voice in the affairs of your nursing profession. Membership in these associations is important to your development as a practical/vocational nurse, and you are encouraged to be active and participate in professional organizations and associations of interest.

National League for Nursing

The National League for Nursing is a large organization concerned primarily with nursing education and improving the quality of health care. It was founded in 1952, and its membership is open to anyone interested in promoting and improving health care through nursing service. The official publication of NLN is *Nursing and Health Care*. The organization provides continuing education programs and conducts one of the largest professional testing services in the country. Because NLN offers individual and agency memberships, it is one of the strongest professional associations in the United States.

One of the divisions or councils of NLN is the Council of Practical Nursing Program (CPNP); it is primarily concerned with practical/vocational nursing issues. CPNP accredits practical/vocational nursing education programs and provides continuing education programs for program directors and instructors. NLN's address is National League for Nursing, 10 Columbus Circle, New York, New York 10019.

National Association for Practical Nurse Education and Service, Inc.

The National Association for Practical Nurse Education and Service, Inc. (NAPNES) was organized in 1941 and is the oldest organization dedicated exclusively to practical/vocational nursing. The purpose of NAPNES is to promote an understanding of practical/vocational nursing through establishing and maintaining educational standards for practical/vocational nursing preparation. It provides opportunities for L.P./L.V.N.s to participate in continuing education programs. NAPNES publishes standards of nursing practice, and its official publication, the *Journal of Practical Nursing*, provides its members with information on organizational activities. Membership is open to licensed practical/vocational nurses, practical/vocational nursing students, faculty and school directors, healthcare agency personnel, physicians, and laypersons interested in promoting practical/vocational nursing.

National Federation of Licensed Practical Nurses

The purpose of NFLPN is to promote the practice of practical nursing and is dedicated to maintaining high standards of nursing education for practical nursing. It was founded in 1949, and its membership is limited to practical/vocational nurses. NFLPN was influential in changing the membership composition of state boards of nursing examiners to include a practical/vocational nurse. The activities of the association include defining ethical conduct, providing standards and scope of practice for practical/vocational nursing, and sponsoring educational programs that provide continuing education credit.

Participation in professional organizations and associations can be an important factor in your development as a practical/vocational nurse. Your active involvement can provide opportunities for professional and personal growth through educational opportunities. An added benefit is the opportunity to meet nursing leaders and share ideas about healthcare issues and nursing problems, a process called networking.

MENTORING/NETWORKING

Helping the new graduate practical/vocational nurse adapt to and function effectively in the real nursing world is a responsibility that has not always been addressed satisfactorily. A technique that is used now, especially in the student nurse's final few months of school, is *mentoring*. It provides an opportunity for the student to function alongside the staff nurse in the clinical setting under supervision, but with a higher degree of responsibility.

In the mentoring relationship, the new graduate practical/vocational nurse has access to the wisdom and knowledge of the more experienced nurse. There is general learning of values, acceptable methods of nursing practice, and practical "tips of the trade." When this happens in a supportive atmosphere, trust develops, and the new graduate nurse can easily turn to the mentor nurse for advice and information.

There are several factors that a mentor must consider for a successful mentoring relationship. The mentor should place emphasis on the successes of the new graduate in a congenial and empathetic atmosphere. Criticism should be provided in a constructive, teaching manner. Guidelines for being a successful mentor include:

- Assist in removing feelings of insecurity
- Reassure to increase confidence
- Help to decrease fears

The mentoring process can be a success both for the new graduate and the mentor. The advantages are obvious, and it can be utilized as a worthy method of transition from student to graduate practical/vocational nurse.

Networking is defined as any system of lines or channels interlacing like the fabric of a net. It is the interlacing that makes networking so beneficial to all involved. The system is made stronger by the people participating in it. From a nursing focus, networking is simply connecting with other nurses through meetings, conventions, seminars, workshops, classes, professional associations, and committees. At these various functions, there is an opportunity to share information, ideas, strategies, policies, and a wide variety of common issues. Discussions can lead to clarity and a better understanding of trends and issues in nursing and health care and can be a springboard for creativity and a testing ground for challenging ideas, new ideas that may possibly solve some of the most difficult problems in nursing and health care.

A key to the strength and success of networking is communication. This is accomplished in a variety of ways. The exchange of business or personal cards is a good start. When exchanging cards, it is helpful to write on the back of the card the person's occupation, hours for contact, and their area of interest. Make sure that the telephone number is included since some personal cards do not have telephone numbers printed on them. Keep the cards in a holder in a systematic format. Stay in contact by letter or, if needed, by telephone. This contact keeps you fresh in the person's mind. You never know when a particular contact may prove to be helpful. For example, a graduation speaker, a writer for a lecture on a very specialized subject, a consultant, trainer, substitute teacher, or a referral is often the fruit of a networking contact.

Networking continues to be a strong method of communication between nurses in their professional organizations and associations. This process can provide opportunities for all involved.

POLITICAL INVOLVEMENT

Nurses and legislators share a mutual need. Nurses need legislators to represent their interests, and legislators need nurses' votes.

Developing a relationship with a legislator is one of the best ways to pave the road for access to that legislator on issues critical to nursing. A good relationship with your representative is usually based on mutual interests and needs.

It is up to you to demonstrate that you share interests. This is usually not too difficult. You probably already have enough statistics to discuss the issue in which you are interested and how it impacts your legislator's district. The task is to communicate the mutual interest and needs to your legislator, a key step in political organizing.

The key to effective communication is to know your legislator. The more familiar you are with your legislator, the better you will be able to communicate your concerns in terms he or she can understand.

You will need some background on your legislator, which your professional association may be able to provide. Background information includes profession, length of time in legislature, party affiliation, record on issues nurses care about, experience and history with nurses' issues, and nursing associates.

Legislators ask themselves many questions before they vote to support or oppose a bill. Considerations include:

- Does this measure affect my district, and if so, how?
- Does my political party caucus support or oppose the bill?
- Who are supporting/opposing the bill and what kind of relationship do I have with them?
- What do my major campaign contributors think about the bill?
- What do people in my district think? Have they communicated with me?

How to Communicate: Writing and Calling

Because legislators do not have in-depth knowledge on every issue, they rely on input from experts. That's where the practical/vocational nurse plays an important part. Taking the time to write to your legislator is probably one of the most important steps you can take to protect the future of your profession.

A letter written by a well-informed individual lets the legislator know the writer is serious about the issue. Address the legislator as "The Honorable Jane Smith." Be sure to include your address. Identifying a bill by name, number, and author makes it easier for the legislator to recognize what you are talking about.

Open your letter by identifying your position on the bill and use the rest of the letter to justify your position. When possible, first state how the legislation would affect patient care, then address how it would impact nurses. A personal letter is more effective than petitions or photocopied letters. Do not be rude or insulting or threaten your legislator. Be polite and thank the legislator for taking the time to read your letter. Be clear and concise. Offer to provide more information. Have the facts. Always send a copy of your letter to your nursing organization, so they can keep track of any lobbying efforts made to each legislator.

If the time is limited, your nursing organization may ask nurses to call their legislator to get support on a bill. Calling the legislator's office is an effective tactic at the right time. Give the staff your name, the name and number of the bill, and briefly state your position on the bill and how you would like your legislator to vote. This should take only a few minutes. If you need further information on the status of the bill, or you want to know how your legislator voted, you can call the government relations office of your nursing organization.

When your legislator votes with you, do not forget to say thank you. A follow-up note or call is appreciated. Another important point to remember is that when contact is made with a legislator, it should not always be to ask for something. For example, you can offer to help the staff draft responses to constituent letters that deal with health-related issues.

Checklist: Writing Your Legislator

- Identify the bill by name, number, and author.
- Open the letter by identifying your position and use the rest of the letter to support your reasoning.
- When possible, first state how the bill will affect patient care.
- Have the facts.
- Offer to provide more information.
- Be polite, clear, and concise.
- Send a copy to your nursing organization.
- When your legislator votes with you, do not forget to say thank you.

Sample Letter

Dear Senator Jones,

I am writing to ask your support for SB 1234 by Senator Love. This bill would create a scholarship program for practical/vocational nurses. It is sponsored by the National Association for Practical Nurse Education and Service, Inc., of which I am a member.

The nursing shortage will only get worse in the future unless something is done. The public needs to know there will be enough nurses to care for the sick and injured.

SB 1234 targets areas that lack health care and groups that are underrepresented in nursing. I am proud of the National Association for Practical Nurse Education and Service, Inc. that would make nursing more representative of America's population.

I really hope you can support this bill. This is a very important bill for nursing. If you need any more information, please contact me, I would be happy to help.

My name and address are: Mary Smith, 5678 Elm Street, Pine Oaks, CA 00099, telephone (123) 467-6789.

Sincerely,
Mary Smith, L.V.N.

REVIEW/DISCUSSION/ACTIVITIES

1. State five qualities of the effective nurse leader.
2. What are the two organizations associated with practical/vocational nursing? Discuss the purpose of each.
3. What is the relationship between NLN and practical/vocational nursing?
4. What is networking? Discuss the advantages.
5. Invite a representative from a practical/vocational nursing organization to speak to the class about the advantages of membership and the purposes of the organization.
6. List six important items to remember when writing your legislator.

BIBLIOGRAPHY

Bagwell, M. and Clements, S. *A Political Handbook for Health Professionals*. Boston: Little Brown, 1985.

Ellis, Janice R., and Hartley, Celia L. *Nursing in Today's World*, 3d ed. Philadelphia: J.B. Lippincott, 1988.

Grippando, Gloria M. *Nursing Issues and Perspectives,* 3d ed. Albany, N.Y.: Delmar, 1986.

Kron T. *The Management of Patient Care: Putting Leadership Skills to Work*. Philadelphia, W.B. Saunders, 1981.

Murchinson, Irene, et al. *Legal Accountability in the Nursing Process,* 2d ed. St. Louis: C.V. Mosby Co., 1982.

CHAPTER
10

Career Awareness

The student successfully attaining the goals of this chapter will be able to:

- List factors included in self-assessment.
- List sources of job leads.
- Identify the components of an appropriate resume format.
- Write a resume.
- Write a cover letter or a letter of application.
- Describe the four segments of an interview.

THE CHALLENGE OF TRANSITION

The transition from student to graduate can be frustrating and stressful, sometimes leaving the nurse completely disillusioned. Leaving the protected academic setting of the classroom and entering the real world of practical/vocational nursing can be an overwhelming experience. The new graduate may encounter high and unrealistic expectations combined with an inability to effect positive change. Realistically, all too often one's focus is directed toward getting the essentials of the job done in the time allowed. The new graduate may feel that it is impossible to administer the quality nursing care needed within the limitations of the current healthcare system. All of this describes what our nursing education experts call *reality shock*.

Nurses have reacted to reality shock in a variety of ways, including leaving nursing altogether, returning to school for answers to an imperfect problem, or going from one job to another, looking for "greener pastures," i.e., "job hopping." Some try to "stand their ground" and fight the system and are soon viewed as troublemakers for the system. Still others just give up on their quality beliefs and join forces with the inadequacies and flaws of the system.

The perfect solution does not yet exist to combat the far-reaching effects of reality shock. However, a discussion of employer expectations may provide the basis to review your nursing strengths and to identify those skill areas requiring more study and refinemnt.

EMPLOYER EXPECTATIONS

It is important to take a look at the expectations of the new graduate practical/vocational nurse from the employer's perspective. The expectations may vary depending upon the facility, the geographical area, and various community factors. Generally, employers expect the newly graduated, entry-level practical/vocational nurse to exhibit competencies in the following areas:

- Theoretical knowledge necessary for basic patient care and decision making.
- Knowledge of the nursing process.
- Self-awareness, recognizing skills, abilities, and limitations.
- Understanding of the recordkeeping function.
- Commitment to duties and responsibilities.
- Proficiency in basic nursing care procedures.
- Efficiency in performance of duties.

Let's discuss these seven areas briefly. The theoretical knowledge learned in the classroom must be applied appropriately in the delivery of patient care. Patient care must be given in a safe and therapeutic manner utilizing specific nursing skills. The steps in the nursing process are assessment, planning, intervention, and evaluation. This process must be incorporated in a systematic approach to patient care through the development and use of patient nursing care plans.

Recognizing skills, abilities, and limitations is an expected trait of the newly graduated practical/vocational nurse. Employers expect to provide guidance to their employees, and efforts can be maximized when limitations are recognized.

Appropriate documentation is one of the most important aspects of the nurse's duties. It is expected that the nurse will know what to document; however, the mechanics of the hospital's system may have to be acquired with practice. A commitment to duty and responsibility is necessary, and the employer expects you to support the policies and the philosophy of the institution.

The practical/vocational nurse is required to perform a variety of tasks and procedures. Some of these tasks are basic to the patient's care and well-being. Knowledge and proficiency in these basic nursing functions is important to assure patient care delivery by direct performance or by supervising others. Efficiency in performing duties is vital. It is expected that the new graduate will require a certain period of time for orientation. These orientation programs can vary in length, depending on the expectations of the employer and the current function within the nursing department.

Now that you know what the expectations include, do a self-assessment based on the seven areas discussed here. Determine your stengths and limitations. Talk to other new graduates who are employed and discuss what was expected of them. This will give you a realistic view of current issues. Your weaknesses and limitations can be viewed as areas of focus to be examined with a problem-solving attitude. Remember, even if you cannot solve all of the issues, self-awareness can itself promote growth. This problem-solving attitude may allow you to take a course in a particular subject of interest. For example, if you determine that your organizational skills are not as refined as they should be, a seminar or a workshop may be just what you need.

Consultation with your clinical instructor may be of value. Ask for the instructor's views on your special areas of need. You may ask for assignments that will assist you in resolving the problem. Some students choose to work in a clinical setting part time while still in school to obtain experience with employer expectations in the work setting. Research papers, additional reading, and viewing educational films on varying procedures are all strategies that have proved helpful to students and to new graduates.

The mentoring relationship discussed earlier in this text is a very useful tool. Many hospitals now have internship programs designed to help the new graduate through this period of transition. As mentioned earlier, employers usually have orientation programs for the new employee. As you work in your facility, there will be opportunities to become actively involved, perhaps through committees or an association. Some of these committees and organizations are agents for change and are actively involved in promoting appropriate and innovative ideas for improvement. Become familiar with the system in which you work, and get to know the people involved. Most of all, observe what is happening around you and use your time and efforts prudently.

GOAL SETTING/SELF-ASSESSMENT

Goal setting is an important tool in several areas of our lives. Personal and professional goal setting is a necessary component of guidance and direction.

Important to goal setting is self-assessment. Factors for consideration include strengths, interests, clinical areas in which you are comfortable, work preferences, personal characteristics, health and physical restrictions, successful clinical and professional experiences in the past, your response to supervision, your need for independence or autonomy, your ability to transfer locations and/or travel, weaknesses, family commitments and responsibilities, educational needs, teaching and planning abilities, and limitations.

Once you have completed your self-assessment, write down your strengths, interests, and weaknesses. Discuss this written evaluation with a nurse who is well versed in career planning and nursing education. Include any comments you receive as you rewrite the evaluation. Nursing education counselors and mentors are good resources for consultation.

An essential factor in the assessment and goal setting process is the recognition of weaknesses or areas of focus. Most of us do not like to think about weaknesses, but they do exist and can be used as areas of focus for growth and enhancement, both personally and professionally. Recognizing weaknesses is a strength within itself. It does not mean that you will try to change every recognized weakness, but the recognition can be a springboard for growth in determining future educational needs and can assist in keeping your professional goals on a realistic track. A plan for goal setting includes:

- Identify the goal to be achieved.
- Identify and establish assumptions.
- Consider the obstacles.
- Plan a sequential process.
- Develop an alternate plan for each step of the process.
- Determine the dates for completion of each step.
- Continue to evaluate your plan at periodic intervals.

COPING WITH ORIENTATION PROGRAMS _____

The first-day jitters when starting a new job have been experienced by all nurses. Will I be able to handle the job? Who are the people I should know? Will I ever learn the policies and procedures? What is the hospital philosophy? These questions reflect some of the concerns of the new nurse employee. It is important to remember that you are not alone—for most of us the mere idea of being in new surroundings can be anxiety provoking.

Most hospitals and healthcare agencies provide orientation programs for their new employees. The programs may be run by one or several persons. Sometimes various departments will provide departmental representatives to assist in the orientation process. A few suggestions discussed below may ease the orientation to a new facility.

If it is not provided, request a written job description of your position. Most employers provide a copy of the job description during the interview. Read it over to see if you have questions. Always remember to bring paper and pen with you during the orientation program.

Most hospitals include an orientation checklist covering those items with which you must be familiar at the end of the orientation program. You can highlight or make a special note of the most important or significant items, which you want to refer to later.

When reviewing policy and procedure manuals, review the table of contents to help you find the most important items or those items that you may want to review first.

Some hospitals assign the new employee to a tenured employee for orientation to the particular area. Sharing the work assignment can be very helpful. This provides consistent teaching by one person and improves accountability for the success and quality of the orientation program.

New graduate nurses have stated that some orientation programs are too short or do not cover vital operational information. Some believe there should be more hands-on involvement. Many hospitals now offer internship programs, which are usually longer and more clinically intensive than the traditional orientation program. Clinical instruction is provided, and the orientee has an opportunity to increase skills and competency while gaining confidence in the new surroundings.

The final step of any orientation or internship program is evaluation. There should be a constant exchange of information between the orientee and the nurse assigned to provide the orientation. Evaluation should be given at the end of every shift so that any problems can be quickly corrected. All evaluations should be discussed, and the comments of both nurses should be included. It is important that all evaluations be in writing, to provide for accountability and follow-through. The daily evaluations can then be used to complete the final written evaluation. All documentation becomes a part of the employee's personnel file, and a copy is provided to the employee. This avoids surprises.

HOW TO LAND THE PERFECT JOB

When you are trying to find the right job, you first have to know exactly what it is you want. It's not easy to articulate your goals, especially if you are just starting out. But having career job objectives clearly in mind is the first step toward making things happen. Ask yourself some questions—and answer them. Do it on paper if that makes you more comfortable in organizing your thoughts. Are you interested in a particular specialty? Is a return to school on your agenda? What do you want to be doing three years from now? Five years? Ten?

Then do think about the kind of workplace and community you prefer. Do you thrive on city life, or are wide-open spaces essential for you?

Once you have answered these basic questions, you can take a discriminating look at your choices. When you have narrowed down the choice to those agencies where you would like to work, you are ready to go after a job.

Whether you are headed into a specialty or committed to general nursing, there are plenty of exciting jobs around. The trick, however, is to find the right one. Most of us tend to be uncritical when considering a job. If the location and the wages are agreeable, we simply do not explore other issues, such as the management style of the agency administration and the nursing delivery system—this could mean the difference between enjoying our work and watching the clock. Many nurses discover soon after they sign on that the job is not for them, but leaving jobs frequently can label you a jobhopper. No matter how sharp your skills are, healthcare agencies will be reluctant to hire you. So it is to your advantage to be selective before you accept the job.

HOW TO FIND SOURCES OF JOB LEADS _____

Go to your local state employment development department for facts about job opportunities in your community.

Ask your relatives, friends, and neighbors for information about possible jobs in your field. Visit your school or college if it maintains a placement list. Read the want ads in the newspaper and trade journals.

Contact employment agencies and other organizations that help people find jobs, including posted library listings, recruiters, and job search agencies. The chamber of commerce lists many of the hospitals and healthcare agencies doing business in your community.

Contacts are very important. List all the people you know who are presently employed. Then talk to them! Perhaps they cannot help you directly, but they may be able to give you the names of other individuals who can. One of these individuals may know of a job that is just right for you.

Once you have found these health institutions:

1. Write down their names, addresses, and phone numbers.
2. Call each firm and ask for the name of the personnel director.
3. Send each one a resume and an application or cover letter.
4. Whenever you mail out a resume, follow it up with a phone call.
5. Keep a record of all the people you have contacted. Put down their responses to your letters and calls. Make a note if you are supposed to contact them in the future for a possible job.
6. Show your appreciation to people who have helped you in the job search. A phone call or short note is usually appropriate and generally persuades them to keep on helping you.

RESUME PREPARATION _____

There are three good reasons for preparing a resume, even if your job objective is a staff slot. First, the process of putting together a resume helps you sort through your qualifications in preparations for the upcoming interview. Getting your professional life on paper can also help clarify goals and uncover hidden strengths.

Second, an application asks for simple facts, while a resume can elaborate on those facts and highlight skills and experiences that the application form might ignore altogether.

Last, a resume is the mark of a professional; remember that this quality—or lack of it—reveals itself in every aspect of your working life, from the way you handle yourself at staff meetings to the way you go about looking for a job. Your resume is the first impression your employer has of you. Make the first encounter totally professional. Your resume should be neat, crisp, sharp, complete, and error free.

Analyze Your Skills

The first and most important thing to do as you write your resume is to analyze your talents and experiences. One of the biggest stumbling blocks that nurses set up for themselves is the unconscious tendency to minimize their assets. It is important to get a picture of yourself down on paper, for your eyes only, before you draft your resume. Write everything down, even skills that seem second nature to you. Knowledge and talents that you take for granted may be far above the norm. Consider your outside interests and skills as well. Are you fluent in a foreign language? In some geographic areas, this ability will immediately boost your professional worth.

For each nursing position you have held, you should be able to come up with at least a half-dozen sentences or phrases that indicate your personal approach and extra contributions to the job.

This list of skills will not translate directly into your resume, but it will serve as a bank from which you can draw. Add to this bank your educational history, professional memberships, and honors. You will not use all this information—brevity, after all, is the key to getting your resume read—but you will have it at hand. And what you do not use in your resume could well find its way into the interview.

Resume Format

As for the format your resume should take, keep in mind that the object is to make it as easy as possible for a busy recruiter to read it. Present the information clearly and simply.

Name, address (do not abbreviate), home and work telephone numbers, and your license number should always head the resume. The next section should present information you think is most important in getting your next job. For most nurses, that means professional experience. Start with your most recent job and work backwards, including for each entry the dates employed, the name and location of the employer, your title, and your duties. Follow this with your post high school education, giving the names and locations of the schools, dates you attended, and degrees or certificates awarded. If, however, your newly acquired IV certification is what you feel most qualifies you for a job, you might want to list your educational background first. Similarly, new graduates might reverse the standard experience–education order.

After these three main sections comes optional information, such as seminars attended, honors received, and membership associations. Do not list every professional activity and achievement. Pick two or three that are pertinent to your career goals. Otherwise, you will overwhelm the reader, and some important data might be overlooked.

Do not include community activities, hobbies, marital status, number of children, age, or health status. The information will not help the person screening applications decide if you are qualified for the job, but it will clutter things considerably.

Also, do not include references. Simply say they will be provided on request. There is no point in handing out this information before an employer asks for it. It is, however, a good idea to draw up your list of references, have it neatly typed, photocopied, and on hand.

If possible, limit your resume to a single page. Rarely, if ever, should a resume exceed one page. Recruiters and personnel directors screen dozens of resumes a day, and loading yours with detailed descriptions of what you did at each position is not going to make it easy to get through it. Assume the person evaluating your resume knows what the job entails and direct your efforts to illustrating your special contributions.

You will have more success keeping your resume to a reasonable length if you avoid overblown language. Pepper your resume with action words, such as improved, established, handled, initiated, planned, prepared. These words convey a lot of meaning in a short space.

The resume that lands on the desk of the evaluating person should look crisp and businesslike, as you do on the job. It should be typed on 8½″ by 11″ white bond paper in black ink. There should be no erasures, strikeovers, or globs of correction fluid visible when you finish. Type a rough draft first to check positioning. Leave ample margins at the top, bottom, and sides.

Before you have it photocopied, critique your resume. Is it too long? Is all the information necessary? Is it neatly written and clearly presented?

Sample Guidelines

Personal Information	Include name, address, telephone number. Home and business numbers can be given.
Job Objective	Stated and described as specifically as possible.
Experience	Describe either functionally (by activities performed) or the most relevant experience

continued

that supports this particular job objective. Therefore, go from most to least relevant, or chronologically list your most recent experience first. Use action words; do not use full sentences unless you decide to write your resume as a narrative.

Education

Depending on your objective and the amount of education you have had, you may want to place this category directly after job objective.

Special Skills

Put this optional category directly after job objective if you feel that your experiences do not adequately reflect the talents you have that best support this job objective.

References

Available on request.

Sample Resume

Mary Brown, L.V.N.
3000 Vista Drive West
Toluca, Arizona 80023
(290) 342-5798

Job Objective: Staff Position, Pediatrics

Education: Overland Vocational Nursing School, 1985
Overland, Arizona

IV Certification
Mayfield Adult School, 1985
Overland, Arizona

Certified Phlebotomist, Hully College, 1982

Experience: Pediatrics Staff Nurse
Hillcrest Regional Medical Center
3000 N. Hill Street, New York, New York 00234
1985–current

References: Available on request

THE COVER LETTER

Never send a resume without a cover letter that is every bit as businesslike as the resume itself. That means a perfectly typed letter on good-quality white paper that conforms to standard business format.

Why take the trouble? Because a cover letter contains the most essential information you have to convey—that you are interested in a particular job and that you would like to set up an appointment to discuss it. It is also your opportunity to personalize your resume by mentioning what it is that convinced you to apply to this particular institution and by drawing the reader's attention to the experience you believe qualifies you to do the job. Like your resume, the cover letter is a reflection of you.

The rules for writing cover letters are few but firm:

- BE CONCISE. The three points you need to make—that you are interested, qualified, and available to talk about a job, can be covered in three or four paragraphs.
- BE PERSONAL. Address the letter to a specific person, never a department or an anonymous sir or madam. Make it your business to find out who will be conducting the interview by phoning the personnel department. If there is no one in particular who does the interviewing, write to the director of nursing by name. Never send a photocopied cover letter with the name of the person typed or handwritten in.
- BE SPECIFIC. Always request an interview, suggesting dates and times and noting that you will expect a call or will call yourself the following week to set it up. And make sure you include telephone numbers at which you can be reached just in case your letter and resume get separated.
- BE COURTEOUS. Thank the interviewer for their consideration. Granted, it is a small point, but courtesy helps oil the wheels of amiable professional relationships.
- DO NOT OVERUSE "I." It is best not to start the letter with "I" since its overuse is irritating to the reader. Suggested alternatives include: "My letter is in response to," "With the recommendation of Jane Jones, Director of Education at General Hospital, I am writing in reference to," or, "The supervisory position described in your newspaper advertisement is well suited to my job objective."

Be sure to make a copy of your letter for your files. When it is time to go to the interview, you will need to review the points emphasized in it. You should also write down reminders to make follow-up calls.

Sample Cover Letter

January 16, 19—

Mrs. Judith Smithson
Nurse Recruiter
Jones-Reese Hospital
13065 Citrus Street
Jonesville, Arizona 78645

Dear Mrs. Smithson:

This letter is in response to your ad in the Nursing American Review for the Pedicatrics Staff Nurse position.

My five years of pediatric nursing experience at a 700-bed regional medical center have provided me with a background that meets the requirements of the job advertised.

Your hospital's successful research program makes it an attractive organization for career advancement. A copy of my resume is enclosed for your review. I will telephone you within the week to schedule an interview. If you need to contact me, my telephone number is (290) 342-5798.

Sincerely yours,

Mary Brown

THE APPLICATION

Remember, the employment application is used by the employer as a screening device. It may contain questions that the employer will review carefully in order to find a reason to screen out your application. One such question is the "reason for leaving" question, usually in the employment history section of the application.

Here are some examples of *red light words* that may get your application screened out. Try to use *green light words* instead. However, always be truthful. Do not be dishonest.

RED LIGHT WORDS	GREEN LIGHT WORDS
Quit	Resigned
Fired	Discharged
Got into a fight	Personality conflict
Hours too long/short	Not my type of work
Moved away	Changed residence
Not enough money	Financial considerations
Did not like the work	Career change Better opportunity
No car/car broke down	Transportation problem

General Tips

Whenever possible, visit the organization or call and ask if an application can be mailed to you. If so, offer to provide a self-addressed, stamped envelope for the convenience of the institution. The purpose here is to make a photocopy of the application. You can then use the copy to work on a rough draft. Use the copy to make any corrections and revisions before transferring the information to the application to be presented.

When you complete the application for presentation, make a photocopy for your records and to take with you to the interview.

Be sure to read the application carefully before you begin writing. Always use ink or type the application unless pencil is specified. Unless a handwriting sample is requested, printing is usually preferred if the information is not typed.

Never leave a question blank, and remember to use green light words instead of red light words. Avoid lengthy explanations: the employer is not interested and will be turned off. Try to be neat and accurate. Do not answer questions in the wrong place.

If you have held a large number of short-term jobs, do not list them all; lists only those relevant to this type of work or that show a particular kind of skill.

Reference persons can include teachers, counselors, ministers, family friends, colleagues, supervisors, or any responsible adult who knows something good about you and is willing to say so. Always notify the reference to expect a call from an employer. Let them know the names of the agencies to which you have applied.

Sign and date the application. Take the time to check it over carefully for spelling, neatness, accuracy, and completeness.

The employment application is a screening device for the employer and can tell much about who you are, what you have done and learned, how careful and neat your work will be, whether you will follow instructions, and whether you can read and write. It may give the employer clues about possible risks in hiring you by revealing trouble spots in your background. The application is often the first thing about you the employer sees, if it makes you look good, she will want to see you in person; and if it is clear and informative, you may be considered for jobs in the future, even if you are not hired immediately.

GETTING READY FOR THE INTERVIEW

Have all the factual information about yourself ready: address, telephone number, social security number. Be sure to include the necessary papers: licenses, health certificates, CPR card, and other records that pertain to employment. Learn as much as you can about the company to which you are applying. Know why you want to work for this institution.

Dress the way you want to be perceived and to reinforce the notion that you are the professional you say you are. Jeans, corduroys, and casual slacks are absolutely inappropriate, as are sundresses, revealing blouses, sandals, running shoes, athletic shoes, bare legs, and stockings with runs.

THE INTERVIEW

The interviewing process is the culmination of your job strategy. Generally, people who are interviewed are assumed to be qualified to do the job; the question becomes one of finding the most appropriate meshing of personalities. Both the interviewer and the interviewee rely on their communication skills, judgment, intuition, and insight. It is a two-way process. While you are being evaluated, you should be evaluating the position and the people offering it.

Some of the best preparation for the interview is research about the prospective employer. You must be able to show the employer why you will be the best person for the job. Relate your personal strengths and past accomplishments to this particular enterprise. Specifically, tell how you can help solve current problems and function as a valuable member of the agency.

Your resume and cover letter become the written and mental outline upon which you elaborate to translate the information into potential benefits to the employer.

Before the interview, verify the particulars. Write down the interviewer's name, the location, time, and date of your appointment. Last minute nervousness can block such details from your memory. Plan on arriving fifteen minutes early.

Take a good look at yourself. Employers are becoming increasingly broad-minded about clothes and hair, but few are totally "liberated." If you are serious about getting a job, then you had better look and dress the part. No interviewer will tell you what you are supposed to wear, but the person will partially measure your maturity and judgment by your appearance.

Before the interview, or early in it, try to find out the essential responsibilities of the job. Make a mental note of them, and throughout the interview, feed back the kind of information from your background that shows that you can handle these responsibilities.

There are some stress questions that you may have to handle; be prepared beforehand with a response that feels comfortable to you. A list of sample questions appears later in this section.

If a question seems inappropriate, you may ask, "How does this information relate to or affect my employment here?" This may prompt an employer to get to the real concerns, such as job stability and commitment to the job and organization. You may even consider bringing up these relevant issues. Seemingly unimportant conversation is often an attempt to put you and the interviewer at ease or to assess your ability to socialize.

Apprehension, tension, and anxiety are a normal part of preinterview jitters. Relaxation techniques and deep breathing may help.

It is a good idea to bring along an extra copy of your resume and references, even if you have already sent them. You may be asked to fill out another application, a task that will be much easier if you can take the information directly from your resume. Also, your photocopy of the application can assist you in completing another application if needed. Additionally, the interviewer may have misplaced the resume you mailed, so it is best to have a backup. This makes you look prepared and organized.

When you meet the interviewer, be friendly, but not familiar. Greet the person by name, look him in the eye and thank him for seeing you. Do not sit down until asked, and do not smoke even if you are given approval to do so. Gum chewing is absolutely inappropriate.

It is important to note that many interviewers are just as nervous about the process as you. Feel free to make first attempts to "break the ice"; while trying to relieve another's anxiety, yours becomes secondary. Note the office decor, the cordial welcome, whatever makes sense as an icebreaker.

Relax in your chair, a rigid posture reinforces your tenseness. Actually, a slightly forward position with head erect indicates interest and intimacy. Maintain eye contact. In answering questions, use your knowledge of yourself to transmit the idea that you are the best person for the job; allow strengths such as good will, flexibility, enthusiasm, and a professional approach to surface. On an index card, note your strengths or key selling points, any questions you may have, and some key words like ''smile,'' ''speak up,'' and ''relax'' and refer to them from time to time, especially just before you go into the interview. Forthright statements about what you do well, with examples of accomplishments, are important. Talk with pride, honesty, and confidence about your accomplishments and your potential, your interest and commitment, and your readiness to learn on the job.

Interview Breakdown

Although every interview is different, most follow a general pattern. A typical half-hour session can be roughly divided into four segments:

1. The first five minutes are usually devoted to establishing some rapport and opening the lines of communication. Instead of wondering why the interviewer is taking valuable time chatting about the weather, your parking problems, etc., relax and enjoy the conversation. The deeper subjects will come soon enough. The interview begins the moment you introduce yourself and shake hands. Do not discount this initial period. Your ability to converse, expressing yourself intelligently, is being measured.

2. The adept interviewer will move subtly from a casual exchange to a more specific level of conversation. The second part of the interview gives you a chance to answer some ''where, when, and why'' questions about your background, to supply information left out of your resume. Now is the time to describe some extracurricular activities or work experience that may explain your less-than-perfect GPA. Or talk of changes effected by you as president of a campus organization or community group. This is your chance to elaborate upon your strong points and maximize whatever you have to offer. Do not monopolize the conversation; let the interviewer lead. But do not confine your statements to petrified monosyllables.

  The interviewer will be interested not only in what you say, but how you say it. As important as the information you communicate, is evidence of a logical organization and presentation of thoughts. Your intelligence, leadership potential, and motivation are being mentally graded.

3. Part three begins when the interviewer feels he has identified your skills and interests and can see how they might fit into the organization. If a good match seems possible, then you become a strong candidate for the job.

4. At the end of the interview, try to find out where you stand. "How do you feel I relate to this job?" "Do you need any additional information?" "When can I expect to hear from you?"

    After you leave, if you feel you forgot to mention something or there was a misunderstanding, correct or elaborate on these points in a letter or telephone call. Write a thank-you letter to the interviewer, recalling a significant fact or idea of the interview that will set you apart from the other applicants. If you are turned down, consider calling to get information to improve a later interview. "I realize that this is a bit unusual, and I am aware that you have chosen someone else for the job, but could you spend a few moments giving me some ideas as I continue my job search?" You could end up with some valuable leads; it is worth a try.

Interviewing becomes easier with practice. Do not be overly discouraged if you do not get the first job for which you interview. Interviews and even rejections are actually invaluable opportunities to reassess and reaffirm your qualifications, strengths, weaknesses, and your needs.

In the competitive job market of today, you can maximize your chances of successful interviewing by doing practice interviews and by being prepared to answer an employer's typical questions.

Typical Questions

There are several types of questions generally asked in an interview. Be prepared beforehand with your answers.

1. *Tell me about yourself.* Refer mentally to your resume; do not assume that the interviewer has even read it.

2. *Why do you want this job? Why did you apply here?* Refer to the information about this job and this institution that makes it particularly appealing to you. Do not give the impression that you are here just because there is a job opening. Refer to the agency's history and reputation.

3. *Why should I hire you?* My skills, experiences, positive attitude, and enthusiasm make me the best person for the job. My personal and professional goals are supportive of the philosophy of this organization. With my qualifications and background, I believe that I will be an asset to your hospital.

4. *What are your career plans? Where do you see yourself years from now?* Employers generally like to think you will be with them forever;

you cannot make promises, but you can indicate you would like to be with an organization that allows you to grow and assume more responsibility and that challenges you continuously. That challenges them to be that kind of place!

5. *Are there any questions?* You might ask what kind of person the interviewer is really looking for. Then show how you fit the bill. You might need clarification on something discussed previously. "When can I expect to hear about the position?" "Oh, yes, I did not mention earlier that," or "I would like to restate" or "reiterate that." Leave the interviewer convinced that you are ready and able to do the job. Never answer a question with "no" without qualifying it positively.

6. *What salary do you expect?* If you have done your homework, you should have an idea of the general range for the position. Never discuss your salary needs before you are offered the job. This is a cardinal rule of interviewing. There are many benefits to a job besides starting salary; opportunities for advancement and training, fringe benefits, good working conditions, good working hours, and so on. Wait until you find out about such things and are offered the job before you answer questions about salary.

Here are some ways you can answer the question: "I am really interested in long-term growth and advancement; right now I am willing to accept your first step salary in the range for this position." "I do not have a particular amount in mind. I am primarily interested in a career with your organization, not just a job."

Or if the interview is coming to a close, and you feel that the interviewer is favorable toward you, you can say: "I do not know what your hospital's policy is, but I do feel I would do an outstanding job for you. Do you have a particular salary in mind?"

If the interviewer answers with a figure, just nod your head and let him go on. He may be offering you the job. Make sure one way or another before you say anything!

In any event, let the interviewer bring up the issue of salary. Do not appear greedy. Remember, you do not have an offer yet.

CAREER PROGRESSION

Now that your basic practical/vocational nursing educational program is coming to a close, careful thought should be given to your future. Serious consideration should be given to your personal and professional goals. If you are satisfied at the L.P.N./L.V.N. level, and this is your career goal, then your educational needs will include updating for currency and learning new methods of nursing care delivery. If you are interested in attaining another level of education, or moving into an R.N. program, there are many educational opportunities available.

A good resource for educational programs is your state board of practical/vocational nursing. The boards are aware of R.N. programs that offer credit for your practical/vocational nursing education. Many state boards have developed progressive L.P.N./L.V.N. to R.N. programs. Some program directors believe that a practical/vocational nursing curriculum can be constructed that articulates with a curriculum that prepares students for registered nurse licensure with a minimum of course repetition. These career-ladder programs are planned to avoid course content duplication and are an appropriate way for students who have the commitment and interest to complete their nursing education.

Maintaining currency of profession is a necessary part of being a nurse. You can increase your knowledge and remain current with new healthcare developments that affect practical/vocational nursing and the healthcare field in general.

The goal of continuing education is to maintain competency in the practice of nursing. In many states, continuing education is voluntary, which means that nurses can choose to take C.E. courses or to not take them without any consequence to their nursing practice. In other states, it is mandated by law that C.E. courses be taken to maintain licensure for practice. In these states, a minimum number of C.E. credits is required for license renewal. Each state is different in the number required, depending on the state regulatory agency.

The basis used to measure credit is ten contact hours per continuing education unit. A contact hour is fifty minutes of an approved, organized learning experience. C.E. program providers offering C.E. programs for credit must be approved by an appropriate approver. This approval verifies that the C.E. program meets certain educational standards. Some colleges and universities offer academic credit in addition to C.E. credit.

Continuing education programs are offered in many forms: staff development programs, workshops, seminars, institutes, symposiums, planned clinical experiences, media presentations, computer assisted instruction, lectures, independent study, and published articles.

If you consider enrolling in a C.E. program, be sure to evaluate the program. First determine your continuing education and skill needs. You may need a certain number of hours for license renewal, or you may want to refine a particular skill of nursing practice. Once you dedide what your needs are, then you can better evaluate the programs offered. Programs are usually evaluated based on purpose, objectives, content, faculty, provider reputation, cost, intended audience, program length, and program approval.

Many employers finance educational programs for their employees. Additionally, you will be respected for your commitment, interest and enthusiasm. After you attend an educational program, be willing to share information with coworkers or to make a presentation. Upon completion of an educational program, make a copy of the certificate you receive to place in your personnel folder at your place of employment. Keep the original for your personnel folder at home. This will be beneficial when you are developing your professional resume.

PREPARING FOR THE NCLEX-PN

The organization responsible for the NCLEX-PN is the National Council of State Boards of Nursing, Inc. The practice of practical/vocational nursing is regulated by states to protect the public from those who are unable to practice nursing safely and effectively. Candidates for licensure are required by boards to show evidence of their ability to deliver effective nursing care by successfully completing a board-approved education program and making a passing score on the NCLEX-PN.

The NCLEX-PN is a one-day examination given in two time periods of two hours each. One two hour period is scheduled for the morning, and the second period is scheduled for the afternoon. Booklets containing the questions and a place for your written answers are provided.

Nervousness is a normal part of test preparation. If you have studied throughout your educational program, and you have achieved success, then you are basically prepared for the NCLEX-PN. Consider the study guidelines discussed earlier in the text when preparing to study for the NCLEX-PN. Additional tips will be offered later in this section.

The NCLEX-PN is designed to measure the abilities and skills required for nursing practice. All of the questions on the NCLEX are multiple choice, and the estimated reading difficulty of the examination is at the eighth-grade reading level. The eight categories of the examination are communicating and participating in plans of care, administering special therapies (medications/oxygen) providing for therapeutic needs, providing for basic health needs, collecting and recording information, maintaing safety, promoting hygiene and self-care, and maintaining a healthy environment.

Test Review Tips

The best study plan is written down so that all needed subjects and items for study are included. Start with examinations, quizzes, and class notes on the various subjects in your nursing program. Be sure to include the nursing fundamentals as a part of your study plan.

Make a timetable, listing subjects in the order you want to go over them. Allow ample time for those subjects you find difficult to understand and for the ones that required more study time during your nursing program. Some educators suggest studying the most diffucult subjects first, using the textbook and your notes for clarification.

Participating in a study group is a good way to study as long as all of the group members are committed to the work at hand. Each member of the study group can lead a review session in their strongest subject, and all members will benefit.

The amount of time needed for review varies, depending on your subject area strengths and weaknesses. Rely on your own study habits if you have been successful with them in the past. If you have not developed good study habits, then you may want to schedule several weeks or months for your review. The important thing is to allow yourself enough time that you do not feel rushed. This preparation is a time for careful study.

Once you have your study plan in writing, be sure to schedule it in manageable parts so that your plan does not seem overwhelming. Make sure you are committed to your schedule and study plan. Plan to end your review several days before the examination. Try to decrease the tension by doing a favorite activity the night before the exam. It is best not to study the night before the exam because it tends to make you more anxious. Schedule yourself a good night's sleep and trust your review and your knowledge of your course material.

REVIEW/DISCUSSION/ACTIVITIES

1. List the steps in the plan for goal setting.
2. Identify five sources of job leads.
3. What are the purposes of the resume? List the parts of the resume.
4. Invite a personnel director or nurse recruiter to speak to the class about the interview process and how to successfully handle the interview.
5. Discuss the purpose of the cover letter.

BIBLIOGRAPHY

Dickhut, Harold W. *The Professional Resume and Job Search Guide.* Englewood Cliffs, N.J.: Prentice-Hall, 1981.

Gulack, R. "Why Nurses Leave Nursing." *RN* 46 (12) (December, 1983) 2–37.

Heschong, Naomi H. *Get the Job You Want,* 3d ed. Woodbury, N.Y.: Barron's Educational Series, 1983.

Lotit, Mary Sue, and Kostenbauer, Joyce. *Advance: The Nurse's Guide to Success in Today's Job Market.* Boston: Little, Brown & Co., 1981.

Rambo, B. J. *Adaptation Nursing: Assessment and Intervention,* 1st ed. Philadelphia: W.B. Saunders, 1984.

State and Territorial Boards of Nursing and Practical Nursing

ALABAMA
Executive Officer
Alabama Board of Nursing
Suite 203, 500 Eastern Blvd.
Montgomery, Alabama 36117
Tel: (205) 261–4060

ALASKA
Executive Officer
Alaska Board of Nursing
Dept. of Commerce & Economic
  Development
Div. of Occupational Licensing
The Frontier Bldg.
3601 C Street, Suite 722
Anchorage, Alaska 99502–0333
Tel: (907) 561–2878

For Licensing Information:
Licensing Director
Board of Nursing
Pouch "D"
Juneau, Alaska 99811

AMERICAN SAMOA
Executive Secretary
American Samoa Health Service
  Regulatory Board
Pago Pago, American Samoa 96799
Tel: (684) 633-1222 ext. 206

ARIZONA
Executive Secretary
Arizona State Board of Nursing
State Occupational Licensing Bldg.
5050 N. 19th Ave., Suite 103
Phoenix, Arizona 85015
Tel: (602) 255–5092

ARKANSAS
Executive Director
Arkansas State Board of Nursing
Westmark Bldg., Suite 308
4120 W. Markham Street
Little Rock, Arkansas 72205
Tel: (501) 371–2751

CALIFORNIA
Executive Officer
State Board of Registered Nursing
1020 N Street, Room 448
Sacramento, California 95814
Tel: (916) 322-3350

Executive Secretary
Board of Vocational Nurse and
  Psychiatric Technical Examiners
1020 N Street
Sacramento, California 95814
Tel: (916) 445–0793

COLORADO
Program Administrator
Colorado Board of Nursing
State Services Bldg., Room 132
1525 Sherman Street
Denver, Colorado 80203
Tel: (303) 839–2871

CONNECTICUT
Executive Secretary
State Board of Examiners for
  Nursing
150 Washington Street
Hartford, Connecticut 06106
Tel: (203) 566-1032

DELAWARE
Executive Director
Board of Nursing
Margaret O'Neill Building
P.O. Box 1401
Dover, Delaware 19901
Tel: (302) 736-4752

DISTRICT OF COLUMBIA
President
Registered Nurses' Examining
  Board
614 H Street, N.W.
Washington, D.C. 20001
Tel: (202) 727-7468

President Practical Nurses'
  Examining Board
614 H Street, N.W.
Washington, D.C. 20001
Tel: (202) 727-7468

FLORIDA
Executive Director
Board of Nursing
111 Coastline Drive, East
Jacksonville, Florida 32202
Tel: (904) 359-6331

GEORGIA
Executive Director
Board of Nursing
166 Pryor Street, S.W.
Atlanta, Georgia 30303
Tel: (404) 656-3943

Executive Director
State Board of Licensed Practical
  Nurses
166 Pryor Street, S.W.
Atlanta, Georgia 30303
Tel: (404) 656–3921

For Licensing Information:
Joint Secretary
State Examining Boards
166 Pryor Street, S.W.
Atlanta, Georgia 30303
Tel: (404) 656-3900

GUAM
Acting Nurse Examiner
  Administrator
Guam Board of Nurse Examiners
Dept. of Public Health & Social
  Services
P.O. Box 2816
Agana, Guam 95910
Tel: (671) 734–2783

HAWAII
Executive Secretary
Hawaii Board of Nursing
P.O. Box 3469
Honolulu, Hawaii 968081
Tel: (808) 548–7471

IDAHO
Executive Director
Idaho Board of Nursing
Hall of Mirrors
700 West State Street
Boise, Idaho 83720
Tel: (208) 334–3110

ILLINOIS
Nursing Education Coordinator
Dept. of Registration and
  Education
320 West Washington Street
3rd Floor
Springfield, Illinois 62786
Tel: (217) 782–4386

INDIANA
President
State Board of Nurses' Registration
  and Nursing Education
Health Professions Service Bureau
964 North Pennsylvania Street
Indianapolis, Indiana 46204
Tel: (317) 232–2960

IOWA
Executive Director
Iowa Board of Nursing
Executive Hills East
1223 East Court
Des Moines, Iowa 50319
Tel: (515) 281–3255

KANSAS
Executive Administrator
Kansas Board of Nursing
503 Kansas Avenue, Suite 330
P.O. Box 1098
Topeka, Kansas 66601
Tel: (913) 296-4929

KENTUCKY
Executive Director
Kentucky Board of Nursing
4010 Dupont Circle, Suite 430
Louisville, Kentucky 40207
Tel: (502) 897–5143

LOUISIANA
Executive Director
Board of Nursing
150 Baronne Street, Room 907
New Orleans, Louisiana 70112
Tel: (504) 568-5464

Executive Director
State Board of Practical Nurse
  Examiners
4201½ Canal Street
New Orleans, Louisiana 70119
Tel: (504) 483–4505

MAINE
Executive Director
Board of Nursing
295 Water Street
Augusta, Maine 04330
Tel: (207) 289–2921

MARYLAND
Executive Director
Board of Examiners of Nurses
201 West Preston Street
Baltimore, Maryland 21201
Tel: (301) 383-2084/2085

MASSACHUSETTS
Executive Secretary
Board of Registration in Nursing
Leverett Saltonstall Bldg.
100 Cambridge Street, Room 1509
Boston, Massachusetts 02202
Tel: (617) 727–3060

MICHIGAN
Nursing Consultant
Board of Nursing
Dept. of Licensing & Regulation
Ottawa Towers North
611 West Ottawa
P.O. Box 30018
Lansing, Michigan 48909
Tel: (517) 373–1600

MINNESOTA
Executive Secretary
Board of Nursing
717 Delaware Street, S.E.
Minneapolis, Minnesota 55414
Tel: (612) 623–5493

MISSISSIPPI
Executive Director
Board of Nursing
135 Bounds Street, Suite 101
Jackson, Mississippi 39206
Tel: (601) 354–7349

MISSOURI
Executive Director
Board of Nursing
P.O. Box 656
3423 N. Ten Mile Drive
Jefferson City, Missouri 65102
Tel: (314) 751-2334

MONTANA
Executive Secretary
State Board of Nursing
Dept. of Commerce
Div. of Business & Professional
  Licensing
1424 9th Avenue
Helena, Montana 59620–0407
Tel: (406) 444–4279

NEBRASKA
Nursing Education Consultant
Board of Nursing
Bureau of Examining Boards
Dept. of Health
State House Station, Box 95065
Lincoln, Nebraska 68509
Tel: (402) 471-2001

NEVADA
Executive Director
Board of Nursing
1135 Terminal Way, Suite 209
Reno, Nevada 89502
Tel: (702) 786-2778

NEW HAMPSHIRE
Executive Director
Board of Nursing Education and
  Nurse Registration
State Dept. of Education
State Office Park South
101 Pleasant Street
Concord, New Hampshire 03301
Tel: (603) 271–2323

NEW JERSEY
Executive Director
Board of Nursing
1100 Raymond Blvd., Room 319
Newark, New Jersey 07102
Tel: (201) 648-2570

NEW MEXICO
Executive Director
Board of Nursing
5301 Central, N.E., Suite 905
Albuquerque, New Mexico 87108
Tel: (505) 841-4620

NEW YORK
Executive Secretary
State Board of Nursing
State Education Dept.
Cultural Education Center
Room 3013
Albany, New York 12230
Tel: (518) 474–3843/3844/3845

For Licensing Information:
Supervisor
Div. of Professional Licensing
  Services
State Education Department
Cultural Education Center
Albany, New York 12230
Tel: (919) 828–0740

NORTH DAKOTA
Executive Director
Board of Nursing
418 East Rosser
Bismarck, North Dakota 58501
Tel: (701) 224-2974

OHIO
Executive Secretary
Board of Nursing Education and
  Nursing Registration
65 South Front Street
Suite 509
Columbus, Ohio 43215
Tel: (614) 466–3947

OKLAHOMA
Executive Director
Board of Nurse Registration and
  Nursing Education
2915 N. Classen Boulevard
Suite 524
Oklahoma City, Oklahoma 73106
Tel: (405) 525–2076

OREGON
Executive Director
Board of Nursing
1400 S.W. 5th Avenue, Room 904
Portland, Oregon 97201
Tel: (503) 229-5653

PENNSYLVANIA
Secretary
State Board of Nurse Examiners
Dept. of State, P.O. Box 2649
Harrisburg, Pennsylvania 17105
Tel: (717) 783–7146

RHODE ISLAND
Executive Secretary
Board of Nurse Registration and
  Nursing Education
Health Department Bldg.
75 Davis Street, Room 104
Providence, RI 02908–2488
Tel: (401) 277–2827

SOUTH CAROLINA
Executive Director
Board of Nursing for South
  Carolina
1777 St. Julian P., Suite 102
Columbia, South Carolina 29204
Tel: (803) 758–2611

SOUTH DAKOTA
Executive Secretary
Board of Nursing
304 S. Phillips Ave., Suite 205
Sioux Falls, South Dakota 57102
Tel: (605) 334–1243

TENNESSEE
Executive Director
State Board of Nursing
283 Plus Park Boulevard
Nashville, Tennessee 37219–5407
Tel: (615) 361–6705

TEXAS
Executive Secretary
Board of Nurse Examiners for the
  State of Texas
1300 Anderson Lane, Bldg. C
Suite 225
Austin, Texas 7752
Tel: (512) 835–4880

Executive Director
Board of Vocational Nurse
  Examiners
1300 Anderson Lane, Bldg. C
Suite 285
Austin, Texas 78752
Tel: (512) 835–2071

UTAH
Executive Secretary and Nurse
  Consultant
State Board of Nursing
Div. of Registration
Heber M. Wells Blds., 4th Floor
160 East 300 South
P.O. Box 5802
Salt Lake City, Utah 84110
Tel: (801) 530–6638

VERMONT
Board of Nursing
Redstone Building
26 Terrace Street
Montpelier, Vermont 05602
Tel: (802) 828–3180

VIRGIN ISLANDS
Chairperson
Board of Nurse Licensure
Div. of Professional Licensing
P.O. Box 7309
Charlotte Amalie
St. Thomas, Virgin Islands 00801
Tel: (809) 774–9000, ext. 204

VIRGINIA
Executive Secretary
Board of Nursing
P.O. Box 27708
Richmond, Virginia 23261
Tel: (804) 786–0377

WASHINGTON
Executive Secretary
Board of Nursing
Div. of Professional Licensing
P.O. Box 9649
Olympia, Washington 98504
Tel: (206) 753–3726

Executive Secretary
State Board of Practical Nursing
P.O. Box 9649
Olympia, Washington 98504
Tel: (206) 753–3729

WEST VIRGINIA
Executive Secretary
Board of Examiners for Registered
  Nurses
922 Quarrier Street
Suite 309, Embleton Bldg.
Charleston, West Virginia 25301
Tel: (304) 348–3596

Executive Secretary
State Board of Examiners for
  Practical Nurses
922 Quarrier Street
Suite 506, Embleton Bldg.
Charleston, West Virginia 25301
Tel: (304) 348–3572

WISCONSIN
Director
Wisconsin Bureau of Nursing
Dept. of Regulation & Licensing
P.O. Box 8936
Madison, Wisconsin 53708
Tel: (608) 266–3735

WYOMING
Executive Director
Board of Nursing
2223 Warren Avenue
Suite 1—2nd Floor
Cheyenne, Wyoming 82002
Tel: (307) 777-7601

American Nurses' Association Standards of Nursing Practice

In 1974, the House of Delegates and Board of Directors of the American Nurses' Association established the development of standards of nursing practice as a priority.

STANDARD I

THE COLLECTION OF DATA ABOUT THE HEALTH STATUS OF THE CLIENT/PATIENT IS SYSTEMATIC AND CONTINUOUS. THE DATA ARE ACCESSIBLE, COMMUNICATED, AND RECORDED.

Rationale

Comprehensive care requires complete and ongoing collection of data about the client/patient to determine the nursing care needs of the client/patient. All health status data about the client/patient must be available for all members of the healthcare team.

Assessment Factors

■ Health status data include:
  –Growth and development
  –Biophysical status
  –Emotional status

–Cultural, religious, socioeconomic background
–Performance of activities of daily living
–Patterns of coping
–Interaction patterns
–Client's/patient's perception of and satisfaction with his health status
–Client/patient health goals
–Environment (physical, social, emotional, ecological)
–Available and accessible human and material resources
- Data are collected from:
–Client/patient, family, significant others
–Healthcare personnel
–Individuals within the immediate environment and/or the community
- Data are obtained by:
–Interview
–Examination
–Observation
–Reading records, reports, etc.
- There is a format for the collection of data which:
–Provides for a systematic collection of data
–Facilitates the completeness of data collection
- Continuous collection of data is evident by:
–Frequent updating
–Recording of changes in health status
- The data are:
–Accessible on the client/patient records
–Retrievable from recordkeeping systems
–Confidential when appropriate

STANDARD II

NURSING DIAGNOSES ARE DERIVED FROM HEALTH STATUS DATA.

Rationale

The health status of the client/patient is the basis for determining the nursing care needs. The date are analyzed and compared to norms when possible.

Assessment Factors

- The client's/patient's health status is compared to the norm in order to determine if there is a deviation from the norm and the degree and direction of deviation.

- The client's/patient's capabilities and limitations are identified.
- The nursing diagnoses are related to and congruent with the diagnoses of all other professionals caring for the client/patient.

STANDARD III

THE PLAN OF NURSING CARE INCLUDES GOALS DERIVED FROM THE NURSING DIAGNOSES.

Rationale

The determination of the results to be achieved is an essential part of planning care.

Assessment Factors

- Goals are mutually set with the client/patient and pertinent others:
  - They are congruent with other planned therapies.
  - They are stated in realistic and measurable terms.
  - They are assigned a time period for achievement.
- Goals are established to maximize functional capabilities and are congruent with:
  - Growth and development
  - Biophysical status
  - Behavioral patterns
  - Human and material resources

STANDARD IV

THE PLAN OF NURSING CARE INCLUDES PRIORITIES AND THE PRESCRIBED NURSING APPROACHES OR MEASURES TO ACHIEVE THE GOALS DERIVED FROM THE NURSING DIAGNOSES.

Rationale

Nursing actions are planned to promote, maintain, and restore the client's/patient's well-being.

Assessment Factors

- Physiological measures are planned to manage (prevent or control) specific patient problems and are related to the nursing diagnoses and goals of care, e.g. ADL, use of self-help devices, etc.

- Psychosocial measures are specific to the client's/patient's nursing care problem and to the nursing care goals, e.g., techniques to control aggression, motivation.
- Teaching-learning principles are incorporated into the plan of care and objectives for learning stated in behavioral terms, e.g. specification of content for learner's level, reinforcement, readiness, etc.
- Approaches are planned to provide for a therapeutic environment:
  –Physical environmental factors are used to influence the therapeutic environment, e.g., control of noise, control of temperature, etc.
  –Psychosocial measures are used to structure the environment for therapeutic ends, e.g., paternal participation in all phases of the maternity experience.
  –Group behaviors are used to structure interaction and influence the therapeutic environment, e.g., conformity, ethos, territorial rights, locomotion, etc.
- Approaches are specified for orientation of the client/patient to:
  –New roles and relationships
  –Relevant health (human and material) resources
  –Modifications in plan of nursing care
  –Relationship of modifications in nursing care plan to the total care plan
- The plan of nursing care includes the utilization of available and appropriate resources:
  –Human resources (other health personnel)
  –Material resources
  –Community
- The plan includes an ordered sequences of nursing actions.
- Nursing approaches are planned on the basis of current scientific knowledge.

STANDARD V

NURSING ACTIONS PROVIDE FOR CLIENT/PATIENT PARTICIPATION IN HEALTH PROMOTION, MAINTENANCE, AND RESTORATION.

Rationale

The client/patient and family are continually involved in nursing care.

Assessment Factors

- The client/patient and family are kept informed about:
  –Current health status

–Changes in health status
–Total healthcare plan
–Nursing care plan
–Roles of healthcare personnel
–Healthcare resources
■ The client/patient and family are provided with the information needed to make decisions and choices about:
–Promoting, maintaining and restoring health
–Seeking and utilizing appropriate healthcare personnel
–Maintaining and using healthcare resources

STANDARD VI

NURSING ACTIONS ASSIST THE CLIENT/PATIENT TO MAXIMIZE HIS HEALTH CAPABILITIES.

Rationale

Nursing actions are designed to promote, maintain, and restore health.

Assessment Factors

■ Nursing actions:
–Are consistent with the plan of care.
–Are based on scientific principles.
–Are individualized to the specific situation.
–Are used to provide a safe and therapeutic environment.
–Employ teaching-learning opportunities for the client/patient.
–Include utilization of appropriate resources.
■ Nursing actions are directed by the client's/patient's physical, physiological, psychological, and social behavior associated with:
–Ingestion of food, fluid, and nutrients
–Elimination of body wastes and excesses in fluid
–Locomotion and exercise
–Regulatory mechanisms—body heat, metabolism
–Relating to others
–Self-actualization

STANDARD VII

THE CLIENT'S/PATIENT'S PROGRESS OR LACK OF PROGRESS TOWARD GOAL ACHIEVEMENT IS DETERMINED BY THE CLIENT/PATIENT AND THE NURSE.

Rationale

The quality of nursing care depends upon comprehensive and intelligent determination of nursing's impact upon the health status of the client/ patient. The client/patient is an essential part of this determination.

Assessment Factors

- Current data about the client/patient are used to measure his progress toward goal achievement.
- Nursing actions are analyzed for their effectiveness in the goal achievement of the client/patient.
- The client/patient evaluates nursing actions and goal achievement.
- Provision is made for nursing follow-up of a particular client/patient to determine the long-term effects of nursing care.

STANDARD VIII

THE CLIENT'S PATIENT'S PROGRESS OR LACK OF PROGRESS TOWARD GOAL ACHIEVEMENT DIRECTS REASSESSMENT, REORDERING OF PRIORITIES, NEW GOAL SETTING, AND REVISION OF THE PLAN OF NURSING CARE.

Rationale

The nursing process remains the same, but the input of new information may dictate new or revised approaches.

Assessment Factors

- Reassessment is directed by goal achievement or lack of goal achievement.
- New priorities and goals are determined and additional nursing approaches are prescribed appropriately.
- New nursing actions are accurately and appropriately initiated.

Reprinted with permission from *Code for Nurses with Interpretive Statements* (Kansas City, MO: American Nurses' Association, 1985).

NAPNES Standards of Practice for Licensed Practical/Vocational Nurses

THE L.P./L.V.N. PROVIDES INDIVIDUAL AND FAMILY-CENTERED NURSING CARE

    A. Utilize principles of nursing process in meeting specific patient needs of patients of all ages in the areas of:
       1. Safety
       2. Hygiene
       3. Nutrition
       4. Medication
       5. Elimination
       6. Psychosocial and cultural
       7. Respiratory needs
    B. Utilize appropriate knowledge, skills, and abilities in providing safe, competent care.
    C. Utilize principles of crisis intervention in maintaining safety and making appropriate referrals when necessary.
    D. Utilize effective communication skills.
       1. Communicate effectively with patients, family members of the health team, and significant others
       2. Maintain appropriate written documentation.
    E. Provide appropriate health teaching to patients and significant others in the areas of:
       1. Maintenance of wellness

2. Rehabilitation
3. Utilization of community resources
F. Serve as a patient advocate:
1. Protect patient rights.
2. Consult with appropriate others when necessary.

THE L.P./L.V.N. FULFILLS THE PROFESSIONAL RESPONSIBILITIES OF THE PRACTICAL/VOCATIONAL NURSE. THE L.P./L.V.N. SHALL: _____

A. Know and apply the ethical principles underlying the profession.
B. Know and follow the appropriate professional and legal requirements.
C. Follow the policies and procedures of the employing institution.
D. Cooperate and collaborate with all members of the healthcare team to meet the needs of family-centered nursing care.
E. Demonstrate accountability for his or her nursing actions.
F. Maintain currency in terms of knowledge and skills in the area of employment.

Index